Women and Mental Health:
The Middle East Case

Critical Studies in Socio-Cultural Diversity

Editor-in-Chief: Dr Sara Ashencaen Crabtree

Practice Research in Nordic Social Work: Knowledge production in transition
Edgar Marthinsen and Ilse Julkunen (Editors)

Rainforest Asylum
The enduring legacy of colonial psychiatric care in Malaysia
Sara Ashencaen Crabtree

Men and Masculinities in Europe (2nd edition)
Keith Pringle, Jeff Hearn, Harry Ferguson,Dimitar Kambourov, Voldemar Kolga, Emmi Lattu, Ursula Müller, Marie Nordberg, Irina Novikova,Elzbieta Oleksy, Joanna Rydzewska (Editors)

Active Ageing?: Perspectives from Europe on a vaunted topic
Maria Luisa Gomez Jimenez and Jonathan Parker (Editors)
(SOCNET98 volume one)

The Cup, The Gun and The Crescent: Social welfare and civil unrest in Muslim societies
Sara Ashencaen Crabtree, Jonathan Parker & Azlinda Azman (Editors)

For Better or Worse: Marriage and family in Sarawak
Hew Cheng Sim (Editor)

Diversity and the Processes of Marginalisation and Otherness: A European perspective
Sara Ashencaen Crabtree (Editor)
(SOCNET98 volume two)

Methods and methodologies of social work: Reflecting professional interventions
Christian Spatscheck, Sara Ashencaen Crabtree, and Jonathan Parker (Editors)
(SOCNET98 volume three)

Women and Mental Health: The Middle East Case

Alean Al-Krenawi

Whiting & Birch
MMXX

Published by Whiting & Birch Ltd,
Forest Hill, London SE23 3HZ

ISBN: (print) 9781861776181

Women and Mental Health: The Middle East Case

Dedication

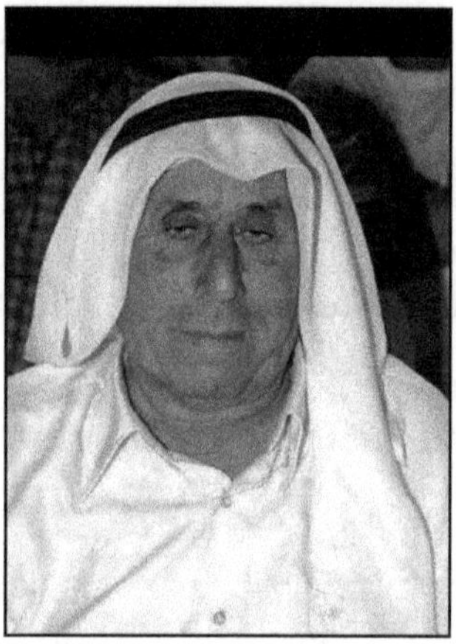

This book is dedicated to my father
Theep Al-Krenawi
Whose life and words of wisdom
And whose understanding of and respect
For all people
Serve as a guidepost
For my life and career

and
To my family
Dr. Monowar, Liali and
Muhammad Al-Krenawi
For their inspiration and support

Preface

Inquiry into the mental health of women in the Arab regions is coming into its own. Mirroring the slow start of gendered investigations of emotional health globally and hampered by the parallel infancy of general considerations of mental health in the Islamic world, serious academic attention finally is being paid to how women in these regions manage their considerable psychological strain.

The author has been at the vanguard of this analysis. For two decades, he has engaged in the treatment and study of Arab women. Already in the early 1990s, the author was combining his clinical skills and knowledge of local ways of being to create novel strategies for intervention with a highly resistant population: multi-unit Bedouin-Arab families in southern Israel. Work with these deeply traditional clients tested the clinical ingenuity of any practitioner, and set the author on a firm path toward seeking the stressors, needs and coping tools of women in this group. At the same time, the author's investigative lens took into its sights the mental health of Arab/Islamic women throughout the world. Indeed, he has found that, thanks to the strong hold of tradition on the Arab populations worldwide, much of benefit may be extrapolated from research among specific population samples in Israel and the Arab world.

And so, the author has continued on his mission: to enrich the knowledge base of the mental health of women in the Arab/Islamic world. The broader scientific community, for its part, has begun to pay heed to this crucial inquiry. Thus we come to this volume. Herein are represented cutting-edge investigations on women's mental health in the Arab regions, and how that health is intertwined with their physical well-being. Moreover, the brand-new field of the social ecology of resilience offers promise for women's treatment in this region, and the author herein presents his tripartite 'Wrap-Around Resilience' program representing a fusion of his research findings and social ecology. Last, the author's life-long commitment to blending traditional and bio-medical approaches has been taken up in full measure by thought-leaders of the medical world, culminating in a World Health Organization prioritization of traditional health strategies. Indeed, progress is being made. And so much remains to be done.

Alean Al-Krenawi, PhD
Professor
Ben-Gurion University of the Negev

Chapter 1
Arab Society

Introduction

'...look and listen carefully, think hard about the big picture, and take responsibility.' *Do Muslim Women Need Saving?* – Lila Abu-Lughod

At first blush, an anthropology-driven admonition might seem like an odd way to open a text on Arab women's mental health in the Middle East. It is certainly a unique way to do so. But Abu-Lughod's sensitive suggestion for meeting the other echoes neatly the tenor of this work. In these pages, we train our sights on women's mental health around the world, seeking the larger, transcultural picture, and then narrow the aperture to view the states of women's mental health in Arab societies. While doing so, we attempt to look and listen carefully, noticing specific ways in which women communicate about 'their bodies and themselves.' Indeed, we shall discover that for women worldwide, body-talk is prevalent, pertinent, and powerful.

Toward the overall goal of cultural contextualization, chapter one sketches, in both broad and more nuanced strokes, Arab societies in the Middle East. Here, we will gain a sense of the geographical, educational, governmental and religious structures in the region. Next, four main elements of life in the Arab region will be noted: constructions of selfhood, Arabism/pan-Arabism, patriarchy and authoritarianism. The hotly contested issue of Arabism will be explored, with an eye toward grasping the different viewpoints on the topic. Patriarchy and authoritarianism, not unique to the Arab world, will be introduced in their particular Middle Eastern forms. A specific form of patriarchy, identified early on by Suad Joseph in her work with Lebanese Arab families, will be presented; this aspect of patriarchy is considered by Joseph and others to drive the institution, accounting for its notable persistence in the region. We conclude the chapter with a review of civil society, and what has been assessed as its failure to eradicate authoritarianism in the Middle East and North Africa (MENA) area.

Chapter two offers a reading on the emotional pulse of women throughout the world. The prevalence of affective disorders rank high in global disease burden, and a review of depression and anxiety among women will be presented. Next, we will discuss the mental health of female children, with a review of emotional distress among under-served populations. Moving to the other end of the life course, the chapter continues with a consideration of mental health among aging women. And, as emotional distress hardly occurs in a vacuum, but rather is influenced by an array of stressors, we will examine how a range of types of violence against women (VAW) takes a massive and growing toll on the mental health of women everywhere. Considered in this section are global manifestations of VAW such as intimate partner violence (IPV), dowry death (bride burning), female infanticide, rape, female trafficking, so-called 'honor crimes' including 'honor murders,' female genital cutting/mutilation (FGC/M), and early/forced marriage.

In chapter three, we arrive at the heart of the book, Arab women's mental health in the Middle East. The prevalence of depression and anxiety among Arab women in the Arab region is discussed, as well as some problems in differential diagnosis of the affective disorders. An account of comorbidity in the Middle East will be offered, highlighting some recent, ground- breaking population studies that shed light on depression and chronic illness, as well as on the possible mediating effects of gender on physical impairment. Deepening the discussion that is broached in chapter one, here we will engage with the ways in which patriarchy, constructions of honor and construals of shame and stigma in the Arab world impact on Arab women's mental health. Case examples will illustrate the complexity of this impact. The topics touched upon in chapter two pertaining to global VAW will be addressed in the specific context of the Arab Middle East: 'honor-based' crimes of violence, IPV, early/forced marriage, and FGM/C. Some similarities will be noted, as well as differences related to Islamic/Arab cultural lifestyle and traditions. For instance, VAW in the Arab home can often take the form of extended family violence toward women, with parents, siblings and co-wives abetting and/or perpetrating the violence. Moreover, VAW (as well as divorce and polygyny) can be triggered in this society by infertility and/or perceived female inability to produce male children. In this section, we also make a very exploratory attempt to tease out the impact of aspects of Islamic religion and culture on the mental health of Arab women. Toward this goal, we review a range of Islamic interpretations on wife beating, aiming to grasp how core Islamic texts deal with this topic. After that, polygyny, which in Islam is permitted under certain conditions, is discussed, with an emphasis on the threat of polygyny around issues of male marital discontent. Finally, FMG/C, which is not discussed in central Islamic texts but is highly prevalent in Islamic communities in the MENA area, is explored. A case example is brought to bear, with suggestions for the clinical management of this extremely delicate topic.

As is true for many traditional societies, as well as, to a more limited extent, less-traditional communities, the mental health of Arab women in the Middle East is highly interwoven with issues of somatization and somatic symptom reporting. Our findings on somatization behavior among Bedouin in the southern region of Israel contribute to a current and heated global discourse on somatization. Thus, in chapter four we take up this topic of current scholarly interest, noting first the nosological debate and its outcome in the newest edition of the Diagnostic and Statistical Manual of the American Psychological Association (DSM-5). This issue has made recent headlines in the broader field of mental health: urged by Kirmayer and colleagues such as Richard Mayou and Joel Dimsdale, DSM-5 provides an utterly overhauled classification of this disorder. Starting in full force with Kleinman in the 1970s and continuing with scholars such as Barsky, Allen and Creed, a great deal of scholarly attention has been paid to somatization behavior, and in this chapter we present some of this work. Honing in on somatization among Arab populations in the Middle East, on one end of the chronological spectrum we have the watershed studies of Lebanese psychiatrist John Racy, who wrote specifically of somatization among Saudi women, and on the other end the recent, massive prospective cross-sectional work of Abdulbari Bener. Somatization across cultures is surveyed next, as well as the prevalence of somatization behaviors in primary care settings. Somatization and affective disorders are then considered, with a review of how affective disorders and somatization affect women in low- to middle-income countries (LMIC).

Moving to chapter five, *The Somatic Thread*, we engage with the notions of idioms of distress, metaphors and proverbs. These three expressive modes are highly imbricated, and the chapter will detail how each has been used by individuals throughout the world to communicate psychosocial distress, often clothed in somatic form. Specifically, we discuss the concept of idioms of distress, coined in the 1970s by the medical anthropologist Mark Nichter, and how he most recently situated the notion squarely within the body, that is, in the context of sensorial anthropology. Next, we take up metaphors, and consider how metaphor may function as the smoothest conduit of illness expression. We then show how proverbs are intrinsic to the daily life of ethnic Vietnamese people, and how their use of proverbs reveals a high level of psychological acuity. The chapter ends with an analysis of the ways in which ethnic Arab women in the Middle East use proverbs and somatic metaphors to convey sentiments about their lives. In these sentiments, which are generally culturally unacceptable to express directly, we can discern the lineaments of many of the stressors addressed throughout this volume. Thus, metaphor and proverb represent for these women a way to say the forbidden. As we will see in the next chapters, the communication of the hard-to-express is the general work of metaphor, but of somatic metaphor in particular.

Meanwhile, *Diviners and Diagnosticians,* chapter six, opens with spirit possession, the metaphor-laden idiom of distress prevalent in Islamic societies. From there we move to traditional and biomedical approaches to clinical intervention for women in the Arab world. This is a complex issue in the MENA area, where, far from being side-stepped or outmoded, traditional healing beliefs and practices remain the treatment of choice – and sometimes the sole available treatment – for many individuals. A recent study investigating the attendees of traditional healing practices in eastern Uganda, for instance, noted that a massive 60-80% of health care needs in developing countries are provided by traditional healers (Abbo, Ekblad, Waako, Okello, Muhwezi,, & Musis, 2008, p.2). Beginning then with the 'diviners,' the chapter explores the nature and types of traditional practices available, considering at the same time how these healing mechanisms tend to be congruent with Arab/Islamic philosophies of living. Continuing the chapter with the 'diagnosticians,' we review a range of biomedical techniques, showing how some, especially the directive, short-term and family-focused ones, may be fashioned into tools that can be used with efficacy in the Arab region. Emphasizing the critical use of culturally consonant therapeutic techniques, we conclude by suggesting that family-based treatment that begins with joining with the authority figure (usually the father), metaphor therapies, and some integrated eastern/western techniques such as mindfulness training (recently rigorously investigated for treatment of somatic symptom disorders) can be part of the therapeutic toolkit in the Arab Middle East.

Chapter seven, *Women of Somatic Metaphor,* consists of three parts. In Part I, the reader is introduced to lyrical somatic metaphor use among the Awlad Ali Bedouin, cultural cousins of the Bedouin-Arab of the Negev. *Ghinnawas,* literally, 'little songs,' are central to a brief exploration of the female management of sentiment among that population. Part II offers a short sketch of life among Bedouin-Arabs in southern Israel, tracing the economic, social and cultural constructions among that sector. The main section of the chapter presents our research on somatization and symptom reporting among Bedouin-Arab women in the Negev. There, we describe a three-stage study in which a total of 525 women from the southern Israeli town of Rahat participated. Both quantitative and qualitative methods were employed in an effort to optimally capture the experience of primary care facility use, as well as differences between married, divorced, widowed and single women in this population. Three main findings emerged from the research: a heavy use of primary care facilities for emotional distress; a tendency toward somatic symptom reporting/somatization; and a marked expression of distress on the part of divorced women, as compared to married women in the sample. These results are contexualized and further considered in chapter eight, where a transcultural synthesis of the findings is offered and a treatment regimen is proposed.

In chapter eight, I discuss the results of my research among Bedouin-Arab women. I found that idioms such as metaphors and proverbs constitute the key to the phenomenological world of the sector, and point to a potent treatment modality. This emic approach serves very well when we consider psychotherapeutic work among the wider Arab female population in the Middle East, and covers some ground too when we look outward at some of the transcultural work that has been done on this intriguing and as-yet-understudied topic. Finally, my work with the Negev Bedouin has yielded insights into the phenomenon of somatization, and in particular, the ways in which Arab women in the MENA region tend to somatize their distress. To recall, these concern primary care utilization, somatic expressions of distress, and high levels of distress among divorced Arab women.

On the basis of my findings, I offer a novel approach to meeting the mental health needs of women in the Middle East. This program, which I call 'Wrap-Around Resilience,' implements cutting-edge work in the burgeoning field of resilience.

Resilience has been described as 'a conceptual nameplate for a strengths-based focus on thriving and positive development among child and family populations at risk' (Ungar, 2010, p.1). Here, I incorporate the newest branch of resilience scholarship, 'ecological resilience,' within the orbit of intervention in the Arab world. The social ecology of resilience, an outgrowth of several decades of resilience research that centered on '...resilience as something individuals *have*, rather than as a *process* that families, schools, communities and governments facilitate' (Ungar, 2013, p. 1) differs from its stock in that it shifts the focus to 'negotiation and navigation' (Ungar, 2011, p. 10).

The principle of negotiation and navigation of resources is well suited to the Middle East context, where persons function within a *sociocentric* (see chapter 1) universe. In other words, in an environment that emphasizes familial, communal and tribal interrelatedness, indeed, where these connections are the warp and woof of daily life, using ecological resilience as a basis for intervention makes a great deal of sense. As well, this direction is in line with Amering's (2010) notion of *trialog*, that is, 'triadic interactions and partnerships among patients, families and clinicians' (cited in Mezzich, Salloum, Ihsan, Cloninger & Salvador-Carulla, 2010, p. 705). Ungar (2011) writes of the importance of resource provision meaningfulness. The proposed program, taking into account as it does the promotion of culturally competent resilience-enhancing resources, answers that call in the context of the Middle East.

In the concluding chapter, we return to important transcultural thought leaders. The overall thrust of this volume follows in the footsteps of giants. Alexander Leighton and his wife Jane Murphy blazed the psychiatric transcultural trail in the 1940s, 1950s and 1960s with their pioneering epidemiological work, the fruit of which inspired the likes of P.M. Yap, Ari Kiev, Arthur Kleinman, Morton Beiser, and Laurence J. Kirmayer. These seminal theorists in turn have seeded the mental health ground with anthropological insight, and are driven to pierce the 'veil of culture to glimpse the shared anxieties, aspirations, and hopes that transcend the gloss applied by culture' (Beiser, 2003, p. 158).

Moving to an alternative, and specifically woman-directed discourse on 'veiling' we know from the penetrating and transdisciplinary work of thinkers such as anthropologist Abu-Lughod, philosopher Martha Nussbaum, and Islamic scholar Leila Ahmed the error of equating veiling with lack of agency. We foreground women's agency in several of the chapters of this volume, aiming to better understand the emotional lives of Arab women in the Middle East, and the context in which female agency functions there. The accent here is on the plurality of *lives*, as the Middle East does not constitute a stage upon which a stock Arab woman character plays her assigned role. We shall endeavor to make use of 'heteroglossia,' as literary scholar Dohra Ahmad has put it in her trenchant reading of the reception of contemporary non-fiction works on Muslim women, in which certain texts, by presenting multiple voices, '...prevent their audiences from generating a single and representative "Muslim woman"' (2009, p. 126). Instead, we shall find Arab women living in geographically, economically and religiously diverse Arab societies that are in the midst of multiple processes and stages of change.

Looking forward, in our conclusion we will assess the directions in which we as practitioners imagine ourselves moving toward the goal of better understanding women in the Arab world, and of assisting them in making mental health gains that work with and not against their specific cultural frames. Fortified by the fruitful knowledge interpenetration begun by the pioneers in transcultural work, we suggest that we continue to learn from, rather than replicate, the ethnocentric-driven mistakes of prior generations of researchers and scholars.

We break new ground in the specificity of our inquiry – to date, the issue of the mental health of Arab women in the Middle East has not been treated in book-length form. We will learn that women throughout the world and in the Arab region in particular suffer from deeply embedded cultural and institutional violence that wreaks havoc with their mental health. As clinicians, we naturally hone in on the suffering of the individual. However, there is a risk:

There is a danger that focusing attention on mental health needs only serves to divert attention from more difficult social problems that demand political and economic solutions. Psychiatry may collude with those who benefit from the status quo, neutralizing political challenges by reframing problems as aspects of individual mental health and offering treatment to individuals who are, after all expressing the pain of a system out of joint (Kirmayer, 2008, p. 138).

Evidence of systemic 'disjointedness' is ample in the following pages, and we will signal some ways in which we may make a modest contribution to its 'realignment.' In all this, however, we will endeavor to be mindful of the complexity of the human condition, and:

> ...concerned with the manner in which human beings – and the cultures they dynamically and interactively construct and reproduce – give rise to 'culturally constituted persons' who are both producers and products of the internal worlds they inhabit (Shweder, 1991, cited in Gone and Kirmayer, 2010, p. 79).

Taking up this pragmatic and positive attitude, we now turn to chapter one, *The Arab World: General Characteristics.*

Chapter 2
The Arab World: General Characteristics

Overview

In this opening chapter, we will review the basic structures of life in the Middle East: geography, language, religion, literacy and governmental and economic structures. Next, current trends for women in the MENA region are sketched. Finally, we consider in some depth four constitutive elements of daily Arab life: configurations of personhood, notions of Arabism, patriarchy and authoritarianism. These four elements were chosen for the strength of impact each has on the lived experience of Arab persons in the MENA area.

Geography

The Middle East is a vast region that is commonly understood to include most of southwestern Asia and northern Africa. Numbering more than 350 million people, the Middle Eastern states include: Algeria, Bahrain, Comoros, Djibouti, Egypt, Iran, Iraq, Israel, Palestinian Authority, Jordan, Kuwait, Lebanon, Libya, Mauritania, Morocco, Oman, Qatar, Saudi Arabia, Sudan, Syria, Tunisia, Turkey, the United Arab Emirates (UAE) and Yemen.

Arabs, Persians and Turks make up the largest ethnic groups in the Middle East. Strong minorities include Kurds, Azeris, Copts, Jews, Assyrians, Maronites, Circassians, Somalis, Armenians, Tuaregs and Druze (Shoup, 2001). Yezidi, Mandaen and Shubak ethnic minorities can be found mainly in Iraq. The Middle East is also home to many Christians, who live primarily in Egypt, Syria, Lebanon, Iraq, Jordan and Israel. The largest Christian populations are Egyptian Copts and Lebanese Maronites. There are also smaller numbers of Assyrians, Armenians and Arab Christians.

Typically, residents of the Middle East have been identified according to ethnicity, religion and/or national identity. For centuries, the word 'Arab' was used in reference to peoples that lived in the northern and central portions of the Arabian Peninsula. As Arab-Islamic empires spread over time throughout the Middle East and into Europe and southern Asia, the term 'Arab' became identified with Arabic-speaking individuals. Indeed, genealogy has been largely replaced by linguistic and political considerations in the identification of being 'Arab.' Currently, approximately 60% of the total population in the Middle East identify themselves as 'Arab' and speak Arabic.

The Arab world spans the continents of Africa and Asia, and encompasses more than 13,000,000 square kilometers. While the terms 'Middle East' and 'Arab world' are often used synonymously, the larger portion of the Arab world is found in North Africa. With eight million square kilometers, Arab North Africa includes two of the largest countries on the African continent: Algeria (2.4 million square kilometers and Sudan (1.9 million square kilometers). Saudi Arabia ranks as the largest Arab country (2,149,690 square kilometers), while Lebanon (10,452 square kilometers) ranks as the smallest land-bound one. Bahrain is the smallest island Arab country (665 square kilometers).

In this volume we shall make interchangeable use of the several common terms for the Middle Eastern/Arab region. The phrases 'Arab world, 'Arab region' and Arab society' are considered by some to be less Eurocentric, and more reflective of the perspective of the majority of the area's residents, as compared to the 'Middle East.' Another phrase we shall employ is 'Muslim world,' which subsumes cultural as well as religious Islamic mores. As more than 90 percent of the region's population as a whole adheres to Islam, much of our discussion on women's mental health in the Middle East will be informed by Islamic/Arabic practices and principles. Finally, the acronym MENA (Middle East and North Africa) is coming into its own on the heels of its use in the context of economic development.

Language

The majority of Arab states hold Arabic as their official language, and a variety of Arab dialects are spoken in those countries.

Religion

Islam, the world's second-largest religion (approximately 1.6 billion adherents), is the official religion of many states in the Middle East. Some countries incorporate within their legal systems Islamic law (sharia). Sunni Islam predominates in the majority of Arab states, with exceptions being Iraq and Bahrain, which have Shiite majorities. Large Shiite minorities can be found in Lebanon, Yemen and Kuwait. Saudi Arabia and Najran have Shiite minorities, and Ibadi Islam is practiced in Oman. Distinctions between the various streams of Islam mainly pertain to views on governing the lives of the faithful, and the role of the imam (spiritual leader) (Pew Research Center, 2011). Arabs make up about one quarter of the world's 1.6 billion Muslims.

Christianity used to be one of the main religions in the Middle East until the end of the 7th century AD. Currently, Christians comprise 5 percent of the population. The numbers are diminishing because of low birth rates as well as high emigration rates following persecution and regional political instability. There are currently about 12 million Christians in the Middle East, but it is predicted that by 2020 there will only be 6 million left in the region. The largest group of Christians are the Copts, who live mainly in Egypt with 6-11 million followers. After the Copts, the next largest group is the Maronites with 1.1-1.2 million followers, who primarily live in Lebanon. The Arab-Christians mainly follow the Greek Orthodox Church and the Roman Catholic Church, with only a small number following the Protestant Church.

The Druze are another religion found in the Middle East. They are monotheists with about 40-50 percent of their members residing in Syria, 30-40 percent in Lebanon, 6-7 percent in Israel, and 1-2 percent in Jordan. This sect is known for their strong self-identity and loyalty among members.

Literacy

According to UNESCO, the average rate of adult literacy in this region is 76.9%. On one end of the spectrum lie Mauritania and Yemen, with an adult literacy rate of just over 50%; on the other end lie Kuwait, Syria, Lebanon and Israel, which boast high adult literacy rates (over 90%).

Youth literacy rates in the Middle East are higher than those among adults. In 2004, the regional average of youth literacy was 89.9% (for males) and

80.1% (for females). Excluding Yemen and Morocco, men and women in the Arab world are basically on par with regard to literacy rates. Approximately the same number of men and women are college graduates (5 million), and more Arab women in this region take degrees in the sciences than women in Europe, according to Middle East analyst Reza Aslan (2013). Nonetheless, a UN survey reported that the average person in the Arab world reads only four pages per year, as compared to the eleven pages read by the average North American and eight by the average individual in the UK. The survey also disclosed that only one new book title is printed per year every 12,000 people. Khalid bin Faisal Al Saud, director of the Arab Thought Foundation, recently stated that slightly more than 8% of individuals in Arab countries aspire to receive an education, compared to 91% of South Koreans and 72% of Australians (Novosti, 2008).

Governmental Structures

Autocracy and lack of democracy currently characterize the governments of the Arab states, which take one of two major forms. Kuwait, Morocco, Oman, Qatar, Saudi Arabia and the United Arab Emirates are ruled by monarchies, whereas the other Arab countries are republics. Many observers view the elections in this region as highly compromised.

Geographical Boundaries

The contemporary borders of many of the Arab states were established by imperial powers during the 19th and early 20th centuries. Major exceptions to this rule include the modern states of Syria and Egypt, which were based on their respective historical boundaries. The newly formed states typically had leaders placed at their heads by these same imperial powers.

Economic Structures

Overall, the economies of the Arab states can be characterized as developing economies. The bulk of their export revenue is derived from oil and gas. This region has experienced significant economic growth in recent years, largely

due to a skyrocketing of oil and gas prices. As well, the recent economic growth is related to a degree of industrial diversification.
The Gulf Cooperation Council (GCC) and the Arab Maghreb (UMA) constitute the two major economic organizations in this region. The term 'MENA' (Middle East and North Africa) region is gaining in popularity as a more inclusive economic-regional phrase.

Saudi Arabia is ranked with the region's highest total GDP (World Bank). As far as per-capita GDP is concerned, Qatar is the wealthiest developing country in the world. The total Arab-world GDP was approximately $2.8 trillion in 2011 (El-Shenawi, 2011).

Current Trends

Women's Development in the Arab World

In 2006, the United Nations Development Fund (UNDF) released a report titled, 'The Rise of Women in the Arab World.' A number of striking points are made by the document's authors, all highly respected Arab scholars. First, they noted that the Arab states have some of the highest rates of female illiteracy worldwide. This and other factors have resulted in Arab women having the lowest rate of registered employment in the world – thirty percent. This in turn has been linked to low living standards and high rates of pregnancy-related disease and death. Two years later, another UNDF report documented that women in this region are denied equal opportunities in a variety of spheres (UNDF, 2008). Further, the authors found that the few Arab women in politics hold symbolic rather than influential positions.

Regarding political participation, Lakshmi Puri, deputy director of UN Women, reported a substantial gap between females in political roles in the Arab world (12% on average) and globally (20 %) (Thalif Deen, 2014). Women throughout the Arab world are behind their Western counterparts in a variety of labor force indexes. Women's participation in the labor force in general in the Arab regions was also found by a UNDF report to be very low (2006). According to Reza Aslan, women's advancement in this region depends heavily on their progress this sphere. He notes Nadereh Chamlou, senior adviser to the chief economist for the Middle East and North Africa at the World Bank, who surveyed five thousand European firms who outsource work to the region. She discovered that while the company representatives claim that they are inclined to hire women over men (they appreciate female 'soft skills' such as dependability), they are disinclined to actually do so because of their perception that *sharia* (Muslim religious law) will interfere with Arab women doing their jobs properly. Aslan concludes that the region's competitive edge in the world market is thus damaged by what he considers a patent misperception.

Nonetheless, there are indicators of professional strides women in the Middle East are making. The increasing numbers of international symposia on these topics that have been organized by different groups (e.g., the Doha International Institute's 2010 'Promoting of Women in Arab Countries,' the 2013 Deauville conference on Arab Women's Leadership, and the Arab International Women's Forum), evidences Arab awareness of this problem. Nevertheless, a massive problem it remains, as set out in no uncertain terms by the authors of the above-mentioned 2006 UN report, The Rise of Women in the Arab World:

This series [of Arab Human Development Reports] has put forward a comprehensive conception of *how a human renaissance in the Arab world may be achieved through the elimination of the region's three deficits: in freedom, knowledge and the empowerment of women.* The vision offered here, and in the earlier editions, is no more than intellectual grist for the forces of renewal in the Arab countries in their efforts to formulate mutually supportive projects across the Arab world. It is hoped that these projects will come together to form a historic initiative to bring the region out of the twilight in which it currently languishes and allow all its peoples to develop and achieve the full blossoming of their potential and a better future for all.

It is also fervently hoped that this historic transformation will be carried out under the preferred future scenario: by taking the path of a complete and vibrant human renaissance (izdihar) (AHDR 2004) based on a peaceful process of negotiation for redistributing power and building a system of good institutional governance. The first act of this scenario should begin with the institutionalisation of respect for the key freedoms of opinion, expression and association, the last being crucial. This should lead to the creation of a dynamic, effective civil society as the vanguard of a peaceful process of negotiation that will avoid the 'impending disaster' scenario of which the Report has warned and whose dark clouds, sadly, are gathering in more than one key Arab country at this time (United Nations Development Fund Report: The Rise of Arab Women, 2006, emphasis added).

The Report details a number of serious concerns vis-à-vis progress in Arab societies: freedom, knowledge and the empowerment of women. These will be taken up in the next sections, as we consider several salient 'ways of being' in the Arab world: sociocentrism, Arabism and pan-Arabism, patriarchy, and authoritarianism.

Configurations of Personhood

In their paper on culture and constructions of recovery, Adeponle, Whitley and Kirmayer, (2012) note that one of many possible conceptions of personhood is likely preeminent in a given culture; for example, a culture may be primarily egocentric, cosmocentric, ecocentric or *sociocentric*. Arab society has adopted the last conception; that is, in the Arab world the

> ...person construes the self largely in terms of relationship to others. The good person is then characterized by values of relatedness, and connectedness to family, lineage, clan, or community (Adeponle, et al., 2012, p. 118).

In the pages that follow, we will see ample evidence of the sociocentrism that drives the Arab region, as well as some conditions that obtain in such a cultural reality.

Arabism in the Middle East

Probing the notions of 'Arabism,' Hopkins and Ibrahim (1997) set forth four reasons for considering the states in the Middle East and North Africa as parts of a greater whole: One, the governments of the respective countries, 'at least on the normative prescriptive level' (Hopkins and Ibrahim, p. 4) describe themselves as units in a greater Arab entity; two, the notion (and ultimate goal) of one Arab Nation is shared across the countries and subgroups within countries under discussion; three, what the authors term 'the passionate engagement of all Arabs in the same issue[s], albeit not with one voice; and fourth, a sociological dimension expressed in migration across country lines for purposes of study, tourism, work, and trade. (Hopkins & Ibrahim, 1997, pp.4-5)

The notion of Arabism has inspired a great deal of discussion across literatures. For instance, Halim Barakat, a highly respected Syrian-born Arab novelist and sociologist, wrote in *The Arab World: Society, Culture and State:*

> One highly distinctive feature of Arab society is the alarming gap between reality and dream. Pan-Arabism is the proclaimed ideal among the ruling classes and the prevailing sentiment among the Arab masses, but Arab society continues to suffer from the erosion of civil life and the profound fragmentation. Efforts at social and political integration have been frustrated by regionalism, the pursuit of idiosyncratic interests by the established ruling classes in separate Arab countries, dependency, colonization, the power of traditional loyalties (religion, ethnic, kinship), urban-rural-nomadic differences, and repressive conditions (Barakat, 1993, p. 3).

Another dissenting insider's voice on the topic, Leila Ahmed has been a strong critic of the notion of Arab nationalism in Egypt and Arab pan-nationalism in the MENA region. Ahmed explores the construction of an Arab identity for Egypt after Nasser's rise to power in her biography, *A Border Passage* (1999). In Ahmed's view, it was only upon Nasser's ascent that Egyptians began considering themselves as 'Arab.' Going deeper into the issue, Ahmed maintains that Arab pan-nationalism does a general disservice by eroding the cultural heterogeneity of all Middle Eastern and North African residents (Thomas & Hook, 2009).

Other scholars emphasize different factors in twentieth-century statesmanship in the Middle East. For instance, political analyst Nadia Hijab, in *Arab Women: Between Defiance and Restraint* (1996) noted that after independence, attempts to construct a pan-national Arab identity that would take into account the heterogeneity of the region ran up against a wall of poor government and bad economic choices.

Finally, we take note of historian Martin Kramer's view. Kramer here addresses the notion of pan-Arabism from the perspective of the renowned Lebanese historian, Kamal Salibi, who critiqued Arab nationalism for:

> ...deluding the general run of the Arabs into believing that the political unity they had once experienced under Islam was in fact an Arab national unity which they have subsequently lost, or of which they have been deliberately robbed (Salibi, cited in Kramer, Arab Nationalism, 1993, p.1).

In Kramer's opinion, this misrepresentation made it 'difficult for them to properly accommodate to the political realities of the present.' Kramer goes on to state that:

> Salibi called on intellectuals to discount the erroneous Arab nationalist view of this history as a united national march that went wrong at some point, and correctly assess it as the parochial history that it normally was: an account of

> so many different Arab regional experiences of one kind or another, fitting more or less into a general pattern. No Arab country today need feel any guilt about accepting its actual existence as a willful or unwillful departure from an Arab national historical norm. It is only when the Arabs succeed in ridding themselves of the highly idealized Arab nationalist vision of their past that they will be able to live together in the modern Arab world as a coherent political community whose various members relate to one another constructively and without reserve (Kramer, 1993, p.1).

We now move to a second main element of life in the Middle East, patriarchy.

Patriarchy in the Middle East

Regarding patriarchy among Arabs, Halim Barakat has put forth the view that:

> ...the traditional Arab father 'has authority and responsibility...expects respect and unquestioning compliance' (Barakat, 1993, cited in Joseph, 1996).

Parvin Ghoraysh (1995) has highlighted several of Barakat's views (1993) pertaining to patriarchy in the Arab world. For instance, Ghoraysh noted that Barakat contended that:

> Arab society...is the family enlarged, and that the family is the society in miniature. Family is patriarchal and hierarchical, particularly in respect to sex and age...(Ghoraysh, p. 261).

Lebanese-born anthropologist Suad Joseph has written extensively on patriarchy in the Arab world. Describing patriarchy in this region as 'resilient,' Joseph deems the patriarchal structure to be a hindrance to the development of states, as well as women, children and families. The researcher contends that the 'persistence of patriarchy' can only be understood within the framework of its full expression; that is, as it is found in the social, economic, ideological and psychological realms. Approaching patriarchy from a novel angle, Joseph takes into account the issues of age and kinship:

> I define patriarchy in the Arab context as the prioritising of the rights of

males and elders (including elder women), and the justification of those rights within the kinship values which are usually supported by religion (Joseph, 1993, 1994a, cited in Joseph, 1996, p.14).

Later in this volume, we will encounter numerous instances in which the rights of males as well as elder women are understood to take precedence over the wellbeing of women in this region. Joseph elaborates on the topic of patriarchy, delineating several types: economic patriarchy, social patriarchy, political patriarchy and self-patriarchy (1996). This last requires some explanation. Joseph is here referring to a process of internalization that she argues constitutes the key to the resilience of patriarchy:

> ...patriarchy in some Arab societies is linked to a 'connective' (or relational) notion of self: a sense of self that is embedded in relationships. In contrast to the individualist, autonomous, bounded, contractual self valued in the West, both women and men in some Arab societies are encouraged to see themselves in relationship to critical others, especially in their families. The boundary between one's sense of self, and other people, is relatively fluid...where a sense of selfhood is fostered which emphasizes the connectedness of individuals to each other, 'patriarchal connectivity' can emerge. This is the fostering of selves with fluid boundaries who defer to males and elders and understand gender and age privilege in kin and religious terms (Joseph, 1996, p. 18).

Joseph (1996) notes that Carole Pateman (1988) has traced what the latter called 'fraternal patriarchy' to European thinkers of the eighteenth and nineteenth century; in this form of patriarchy, the father figure was replaced by the brother. Subordination, then, was construed as male-directed, rather than father-directed. In this way, patriarchy was perpetuated, or, in Joseph's terms, 'reproduced' (p. 227).

Joseph witnessed a compelling example of fraternal patriarchy in her ethnographic work among Lebanese Arabs (Joseph, 1996). There, over the course of a decade, the researcher came to know an Arab family whose brother/sister relationship exemplified the complex dynamics of fraternal patriarchy. As this form of patriarchy is part and parcel of the overarching male patriarchy in the Arab world, and also because our work among Bedouin-Arab women has been highly influenced by its workings, we will spend a few moments now with Joseph's Lebanese family participants, the Yusifs.

The Yusifs were working-class urbanites who shared an apartment in the Greater Beirut area. The family was comprised of a mother, father, five boys and two girls. Joseph's observations centered on Hanna, the eldest son, and

Flaur, the eldest daughter. The passage quoted below immediately followed a scene in which Hanna had slapped Flaur and yelled at her around issues of dress and comportment:

> The relationship between Hanna and Flaur is a prime example of the connective love/power dynamic between brothers and sisters in these Arab families. That dynamic was critical to Hanna's empowerment and masculinization and Flaur's domestication and feminization. Hanna was teaching Fleur to accept male power in the name of love. His family supported his learning that loving his sister meant taking charge of her and that he could discipline her if his action was understood to be in her interest. Flaur was reinforced in learning that the love of a male could include that male's violent control and that to receive this love involved submission to control. She was learning that her brother was a loving protector and controlling power in her life (Joseph, 1996, p. 229).

The cultural canon of male power and prerogative, inculcated extremely early in the life course, affects every sphere in the life of an Arab person. We will see how this canon produces perceptions and expectations that interfere with the mental health of Arab women. Staying with Joseph's work for another moment, however, we see that a further action was being performed in this vignette, one that concerns the *perpetuation* of patriarchy:

Hanna was also using his culturally acceptable control over his sister to challenge his father's authority in the family. By taking charge of his sister, with blessings of his mother and siblings, he highlighted his father's failure as head of the household. Hanna was learning to become a patriarch by becoming a man of the house in relation to his sister, mother, and younger siblings (Joseph, 1996, p. 229).

In Joseph's view, this scenario epitomizes and elucidates a little-understood topic in Arab life: the 'reproduction of Arab patriarchy' (p. 229). As against those who construe the Arab sister/brother relationship in binary terms, that is, either love-based or power-based, Joseph argues for a great deal more complexity. She contends that it is precisely the 'psychodynamic, social structural and cultural processes' *linked together* that are crucial to this 'reproduction' (p. 230).

Suad Joseph's early work has provided a good glimpse of the intertexture of patriarchy and VAW in the Middle East; this topic has been treated in depth by Moha Ennaji and Fatima Sadiqi in their recent volume on gender and violence in the Arab states:

> While gender-based violence is a universal phenomenon, it takes interesting nuances and wears multiple faces in this region where tradition, religion, social norm, war and politics intermingle in a powerful and tantalizing space-based patriarchy (Ennaji & Sadiqi, 2011, p. 1).

The intersectionality of violence against women and multiple processes that are predominant in the current Middle East is afforded an unflinching gaze as well by David Ghanim in *Gender and Violence in the Middle East* (Praeger, 2014). There, the author notes:

> ...everyone plays a part in sustaining and reproducing high levels of violence: men, women, society, the political system, patriarchy and culture. Contrary to popular opinion and media portrayal, violence in Middle Eastern societies is not primarily an external phenomenon imposed by faceless forces of foreign aggression. Rather, violence in the Middle East is a thoroughly familiar, mostly private fact of daily life, an instinct woven into the very fabric of domestic relations. This pervasive, intimate style of violence takes many forms: physical, psychological, deliberate, unconscious, covert and public. The contextual role that endemic domestic violence plays with regard to the notorious societal problems of the Middle East such as the institutionalized violence of terrorist organizations and of repressive autocratic governments is not widely appreciated (2014, pp. xxi-xxii).

In subsequent chapters, we will return to the issue of violence against women, first globally, and then in the MENA region. At this point, we will share the voice of one more scholar, Hiam Salaheldin Elgousi, who has made a current assessment of the power of patriarchy in the Middle East:

By looking to the mechanisms of decision-making processes in MENA societies, it is possible to explain why almost the majority of decisions are taken by men, even those relating to women's issues, when quite simply the answer is: because they can dominate women more and more. *Eventually, the process of controlling women's lives results in the loss of any individuality, dignity, or ability to be independent.* It is also peculiar how, in the process, women oppress other women...i.e., the older women...who have been indoctrinated long enough by men...take active parts in making the younger women in their kin become submissive to male authority in the family.

> It would be almost impossible for a woman to break free from the dictates of patriarchy as any effort to do so would ultimately affect her psyche and will earn her a very negative image in her society, which would affect her self-esteem and status. This patriarchal culture does not just enforce male dominance'

> but also in the process it transforms the whole society into guardians who control the behaviours and attitudes of its members. (in Salhi, 2010, p. 188)

Salaheldin Elgousi is here discussing a multilevel phenomenon, much of which relates to work described throughout this section. She begins with the issue of female decision-making, arguably a 'neutral' subject for which objective observers might legitimately make various claims, and quickly moves to the assertion that the Arab societal norm of men making decisions for the women in their ambit *deprives women of dignity and individuality.* This proposition, taking us as it does beyond the ethically neutral realm to the relationship between patriarchy and women's mental health, will be explored further in the chapters to come. Like Joseph, the author also touches upon the woman-to-woman aspect of patriarchal transmission, a topic to which we will return. Finally, she notes the ingrained nature of patriarchy in the MENA region, and the price an Arab woman would pay for setting herself against this cultural cornerstone. We now turn to a second such cornerstone of life in the Arab world: authoritarianism.

Authoritarianism in the Middle East

In the above-noted Yusif account, we are given a snapshot of how patriarchy functions on an intergenerational level in the Arab family. Inherent to that patriarchy is the notion of a male 'taking charge' of less able individuals, if necessary by violent means. And so we come to the concept of authoritarianism, which complements patriarchy as a governing force in the Arab Middle East.

Eva Bellin (2004) discusses the apparently intransigent nature of authoritarianism in the Arab world:

> The exceptionalism of the Middle East and North Africa lies not so much in absent prerequisites of democracy as in present conditions that foster robust authoritarianism and especially a robust and politically tenacious coercive apparatus. Some conditions responsible for the robustness of this authoritarianism are exceptional to the Middle East and North Africa; others are not...The dramatic transition to democracy that swept sub-Saharan Africa and eastern Europe in the 1990s drew attention to the important role popular mobilization can play in bringing down authoritarian regimes. But the stubborn persistence of authoritarianism in the Middle East and North Africa highlights an equally powerful lesson. Where patrimonial institutions

> are wedded to coercive capacity, authoritarianism is likely to endure. In this context, regime elites possess both the will and the capacity to suppress democratic initiative. And where international support and financing is forthcoming to the authoritarian regime, rapid regime change is unlikely (Bellin, 2004, p. 152).

State-level patriarchy in the MENA region has been discussed more recently in Zahia Smail Salhi's *Gender and Violence in Islamic Societies: Patriarchy, Islamism and Politics in the Middle East and North Africa* (2013). In a review paper, Fatima Sadiqi (2014) wrote:

> ...in highlighting the unequal power relations between men and women that pervasive patriarchy and the rise of Islam exacerbate, the book brilliantly depicts how gender-based violence is sustained by a misinterpretation of Islam, conservative political discourse, and discriminatory Family Laws [sic] in the majority of countries (p. 186).

We will have more to say about readings of Islam in chapter three, but here we will simply note that what Joseph terms 'religious patriarchy' (1996, p. 17) is easily discerned within several of four main interpretations of core Islamic passages pertaining to male engagement with women (see Ammar, 2007, in chapter three of this volume).

We conclude this section with a current assessment of civil society and how the hopes that it would dislodge the Arab region from authoritarianism have not come to fruition. Civil society has been defined as:

> ...the wide array of non-governmental and not-for-profit organizations that have a presence in public life, expressing the interests and values of their members or others, based on ethical, cultural, political, scientific, religious or philanthropic considerations. Civil Society Organizations (CSOs) therefore refer to a wide of array of organizations: community groups, non-governmental organizations (NGOs), labor unions, indigenous groups, charitable organizations, faith-based organizations, professional associations, and foundations (The World Bank, August, 2010).

Paul Aarts, senior researcher for the Netherlands Institute of International Relations 'Clingendael' project, titled 'Saudi Arabia Between Conservatism, Accommodation and Reform' (2012) spoke about the failure of civil society to uproot authoritarianism in the MENA region:

> [...] contrary to optimistic predictions, and after more than two decades

> of civil society promotion, not much improvement has been made and it increasingly looks like civil society is not the force of democratization as it was supposed to be...civil society can be a source of democratic change but it is not inherently one...[...] despite its [civil society's] impressive growth in many countries, [they] have not made a real dent in the region's surprisingly *resilient authoritarianism*...this applies to the Middle East in general...(Aarts, 2012, p.8, emphasis added)

Salient in the above section are contemporary perceptions of 'resilient patriarchy' and 'resilient authoritarianism' in the Arab Middle East. These two modes mirror each other in the emotional status of family and state throughout the region. Shortly, we will consider how they affect women in the MENA locale; first, however, we will take a look at how women worldwide fare with regard to mental health.

> Human suffering is cut from one cloth. Somantic discomfort, social conflict, and existential concerns tend to occur together in the same individual.
> Laurence Kirmayer, 2008

Chapter 3
Women's Mental Health throughout the World

Overview

In this chapter we will review the major mental health risks for women across regions. Depression and anxiety, two of the greatest health burdens for women the world over, will be examined. Next, the somatization to which we dedicate an entire chapter is here introduced. Tackling a topic not yet well researched by the scientific community, we will consider how 'the aging process represents an important variable that exerts a diverse and profound effect on the mental health status of women…' (Malatesta, 2007, p. 2). On the other end of the life course, we take account of how female children fare vis-a-vis mental health. As well, women in under-served populations as compared to women in developed societies are discussed. And, as it is scarcely possible to isolate mental from physical health, this chapter will highlight how the many physical challenges experienced by women and girls the world over directly impact on their emotional well-being.

Burden of Mental Illness across Cultures

A voluminous literature has documented that psychological illness constitutes a major disease burden in both less-developed and developed countries:

Neuropsychiatric conditions are the leading causes of disability worldwide, accounting for 37% of all healthy life years lost from disease; they are the most disabling conditions even in low- and middle-income countries, which may be least able to bear such burdens (Lopez, Mathers, Ezzati, Jamison & Murray, 2006, cited in Wang, Aguilar-Gaxiola, Alonso, Angermeyer, Borges, Bromet, Bruffaerts, de Girlolamo, de Graaf, Gureje, Haro, Karam, Kessler, Kovess, Lane, Lee, Levinson, Ono, Petukhova, Posada-Villa, Seedat, & Wells, 2007, p. 841).

Tackling the problem from the angle of delayed treatment after first onset of mental disorder, researchers from the World Health Organization have noted that, 'Worldwide, mental disorders inflict tremendous morbidity, mortality, and impairment' (Demyttenaere, Bruffaerts, Posada-Villa, Gasquet, Kovess, Lepine, Angermeyer, Bernert, de Girolamo, Morosini, Polidori, Kikkawa, Kawakami, Ono, Takeshima, Uda, Karam, Fayyad, Karam, Mneimneh, Medina-Mora, Borges, Lara, de Graaf, Ormel, Gureje, Shen, Huang, Zhang, Alonso, Haro, Vilagut, Bromet, Gluzman, Webb, Kessler, Merikangas, Anthony, Von Korff, Wang, Brugha, Aguilar-Gaxiola, Lee, Heeringa, Pennell, Zaslavsky, Ustun, Chatterji, 2004); Murray & Lopez (1996) cited in Wang, Angermeyer, Borges, Bruffaerts, Chiu, de Girolamo, Fayyad, Gureje, Haro, Huang, Kessler, Kovess, Levinson, Nakane, Brown, Ormel, Posada-Villa, Aguilar-Gaxiola, Sing Lee, Heeringa, Pennell, Chatterji and Ustun, 2007, p. 177).

The sixty-fifth World Health Assembly, which met in May 2012, detailed an agenda titled, 'The global burden of mental disorders and the need for a comprehensive, coordinated response from health and social sectors at the country level' (p. 1). Agenda Item 13.2 was the following determination of the global burden of disease for mental disorders:

> Concerned that millions of people worldwide are affected by mental disorders, and that in 2004, mental disorders accounted for 13% of the global burden of disease, defined as premature death combined with years lived with disability, and also that, when taking into consideration only the disability component of the burden of disease calculation, mental disorders accounted for 25.3% and 33.5% of all years lived with a disability in low- and middle-income countries, respectively…(p. 2).

Despite this overwhelming attention paid to the disease burden of mental illness, a piece remains missing from the puzzle. Below, we locate that missing piece.

Research Gap

Research on women's health in general, and mental health in particular, lags behind that of men. Malatesta (2007) notes the irony in this:

Women are the primary consumers of mental health services. Ironically, research addressing their unique needs lags far behind that of men's issues. It is only recently that medicine has recognized that women have different health needs and require specially tailored evaluation and treatment services. As a consequence, women are receiving more research and clinical attention...With respect to mental health needs, however, the gender imbalance is more striking. For example, while women are much more likely to suffer from depression, use psychotropic medication and seek the services of a mental health professional, the bulk of available clinical and research studies, until recently, has tended to focus on men as subjects (Malatesta, 2007, p. 2).

In the next chapter, which treats the mental health issues of Arab women, we will find ourselves revisiting the issue of a literature gap. In the meantime, we will approach the topic of women's mental health across cultures.

Women's Mental Health across Cultures

Across cultures, ethnicities and religions, the multiple, often simultaneous roles played by women can leave them at enhanced risk for emotional distress. Women function as daily providers, caregivers to the sick and breadwinners, often for multiple generations. According to a UK Mental Health Foundation report (2014), fully 75% of individuals with emotional issues are cared for by women. Family finances, social relationships, and physical and psychological health can be affected by this caregiving. Indeed, the same report noted that female caregivers are at enhanced risk of anxiety and depression as compared to women in the general population.

Sex differences in emotional illness are a well-documented fact, and, 'it is accepted that women pay a heavy price to mental disorders' (Douki et al., 2007, p. 178). Women are significantly more likely to have been diagnosed with mental illness than are men (29% compared to 17%) (UK MHF, 2014). Sex differences in recognition of emotional distress and help-seeking behavior may contribute to this disparity. As we will consider below, low SES seems to be quite instrumental here, and women are overrepresented in low SES vocations. When women have difficulty seeking help for distress, they tend to turn the feelings inward, leading to eating disorders, depression and anxiety. In contrast, men may externalize their distress, resulting in other-directed violence (Seedat et al., 2009; MHF, 2014).

Somatization/Somatic Symptom Reporting

Women and men differ significantly with regard to both experiencing and reporting of somatic symptoms. In a comprehensive search of more than three decades of literature on bodily complaints, Barsky et al. (2001) found that women, as compared to men, 'report more intense, more numerous, and more frequent bodily symptoms' (Barsky, p. 266). This held true across a wide range of criteria: whether or not medically unexplained symptoms (MUS) were the sole symptoms taken into account, across patient category (medical or community samples) and both inclusive and exclusive of gynecological complaints. Expanding the perspective, these authors marshalled evidence from animal studies that are in line with this data. They concluded that a blend of factors appear to contribute to these findings, including sex differences in recognition and disclosure of distress; inborn sex variance in bodily perception; a sex differential in prevalence of depression and anxiety as well as in instances of abuse and violence. We will now turn to the latter two sets of factors.

Depression

Depression is 'a common mental disorder that presents with depressed mood, loss of interest or pleasure, decreased energy, feelings of guilt or low self-worth, disturbed sleep or appetite, and poor concentration. Moreover, depression often comes with symptoms of anxiety' ('Depression, A Health Concern,' in Depression, A Global Crisis, 2012). The World Health Organization predicts that by 2020, depression will rank second to heart disease as the world's leading cause of disability (WHO, 2002, cited in Ahmed & Bhugra, 2007). Depression is expected to be the highest ranking contributor to disease burden by 2030 (WHO, 2008). Approximately 350 million individuals worldwide have been diagnosed with depression (WHO, 2012). When severe in intensity, depression can lead to suicide, which claims the lives of one million persons per year.

Mental illness is not more prevalent among women than among men, but the former are more prone to depression and anxiety (WHO, 2000). Depression is the 'leading cause of disease burden among women in both high-income and middle- and low-income countries,' with a 50% higher rate of prevalence among women, as compared to men, according to a 2008 WHO report. Indeed, a strong, consistent and worldwide sex differential regarding depression has been found among women and men. Women are diagnosed with depression two to three times more often than are men, and, as with anxiety disorders discussed below, this appears to represent actual prevalence (Barsky, et al, 2001). Grigoriadis & Robinson (2007) determined that this high female to male sex ratio of depression to be 'one of the most replicated results in epidemiology' (p. 1).Thus, as compared to one in ten men, one in four women will be treated for depression at some point in their lives. Post-natal depression has been estimated to impact on between 8 and 19% of postpartum women (Danaci et al., 2002). Depression among women seems to have a seasonal component, as well as being characterized as anxious and atypical in form (Grigoriadis & Robinson, 2007). Seedat et al. (2009) studied sex differences in lifetime DSM-IV mental disorders across cohorts in 15 countries in the World Health Organization World Mental Health Survey Initiative. In all cohorts and countries, women had higher rates of anxiety and mood disorders than men.

Depression, however, can be a difficult differential diagnosis to make. Indeed, under-diagnosis of depression in ethnic minority populations seems to be near-universal. Ahmed & Bhugra (2007) found that depression is underdiagnosed throughout the world in primary care settings in general, and among minority cultures in particular. Bhugra & Mastrogianni (2004) list a number of possible explanations for this phenomenon: variation in explanatory models between practitioner and client; client age and co-existing physical disorder; a variety of barriers between patient and clinician (e.g., racial, linguistic and cultural); doctor's own feelings toward depression; client feelings about disclosure; and not enough investigation on the part of physician for signs of depression. In an investigation of the detection of somatization and depression in primary care in Saudia Arabia, Beck (2004) found that the country's primary care physicians were not skilled at these disorders. In point of fact, the signs of depression are notoriously fickle in nature. Depression can:

> ...hide behind a variety of conditions ranging from accident proneness to sexual dysfunction, it can co-occur.... with a great number of conditions like anxiety, panic attacks, alcoholism and with somatic illnesses like cancer, diabetes and chronic pain. In some cases depression can be expressed with a variety of symptoms other than its cardinal symptom (masked depression, 'depression without depression') and even with antithetical symptoms ('smiling depression') (Christodoulou, 2000 cited in Depression: A Global Crisis, 2012, p.14).

As well, the under-diagnosis of depression has been theorized to be related to issues of stigma (Kilzieh, Rastam, Maziak & Ward, 2008; Kilzieh, Rastam, Ward & Maziak, 2010), an issue to which we will return in the next chapter.

Anxiety

Of all negative emotions, anxiety is considered most universal (Abdel-Khalek, 2004). Nonetheless, this distress category is also highly gendered: across regions, anxiety disorders are significantly more prevalent among women than men. Barsky et al. (2001) pointed to a wide range of studies in which women were between two and three times more likely than men to experience an anxiety disorder. Again, these authors note that this rate seems to reflect true prevalence, as meticulously conducted epidemiological studies report this consistent sex differential.

Writing of the high rate of prevalence of anxiety disorders (from 5 to 20%) in primary care settings, Lasebikan et al. (2012) note that these disorders (as well as depression, noted above) are consistently and globally unrecognized in such arenas. Overall, up to one-third of individuals with mental health issues are not diagnosed with a psychiatric disorder by primary care clinicians (Lasebikan, 2012).

Women's mental health and aging

As noted above, while worldwide, women are the main users of mental health services, the literature is short on research that treats their particular needs. This fact is accentuated by the paucity of work on the mental health concerns of older women (Malatesta, 2007). We shall begin from a linguistic perspective. As they vary with respect to connotation, it is useful to differentiate between the terms 'older' and 'aging':

Older women refers to women age 50 and older. Ageing women refers to the same chronological group but emphasizes that ageing is a process that occurs at very different rates among various individuals and groups. Privileged women may remain free of the health concerns that often accompany ageing until well into their 70s and 80s. Others who endure a lifetime of poverty, malnutrition and heavy labour may be chronologically young but functionally 'old' at age 40 (WHO, 2007, p. 2).

Aging women are a significant, and fast-growing, segment of the world's population. In the fifty-year period from 2000 till 2050, the number of women age 60 and over is predicted to increase from 336 million to slightly more than 1 billion. Most older women live in less-developed states that are experiencing quick-paced population aging. Moreover, the female-to-male imbalance in older age groups increases with age: the oldest-old (age 80-plus) constitutes the fastest growing group among aging women (WHO, 2007).

Depression among Aging Women

Depression among aging women may be related to a variety of life course issues. Examples of these might include a drop in socioeconomic status, bereavement and, as noted above, providing the care for family and friends who are ill (Matthews, Wing & Kuller, 1990; Sorensen, Pinquart & Duberstein, 2002). Older individuals living at home are at a 20% risk of depression, while the risk for those in residential care is 40%; women make up the lion's share of these populations (MHF, 2014). Especially relevant in light of the under-diagnosis of depression in primary care settings, older adults tend to seek mental health care from their primary care physicians (Mickus, & Colenda, 2000, cited in Maltesta, 2007).

A Truism that Bears Out: Variability *Increases* with Age

Malatesta (2007) emphasizes that, contrary to residual ageism-related notions, individual diversity increases with age. That is, countering the idea of lumping together as a sector all older people, humans actually show greater variability in older age than they do in their earlier years. In the view of the author, this fact has real ramifications for the study of mental health problems of older persons. While introducing a series of ten contributions in a volume on mental illness among older women, Maltesta (2007) reviewed the range of papers. Among them, Epstein, Fishcher-Elber amd Al-Otaiba (in Maltesta, 2007) discuss women, aging and alcohol use disorders. These researchers note that the

> number and impact of older female drinkers is expected to increase dramatically over the next 20 years...[and that] women as they age are subject to an increasing physiological susceptibility to alcohol's effects, and

> that women of all ages are at higher risk for negative physical, social and psychological consequences associated with 'at risk' and higher levels of alcohol consumption (p. 7).

Dickerson (in Malatesta, 2007) treats the topic of schizophrenia among older women. She writes that while approximately 67% of men and women who experience a particular disorder as a young adult develop schizophrenia by the age of 40, women tend to experience the onset of schizophrenia several years later than their male counterparts, and that most of the late onset cases are women. Specific gender differences in the prevalence and incidence of anxiety disorders among older women are identified by Weissman and Levine (in Malatesta, 2007). Franco (in Malatesta, 2007) studies post traumatic stress disorder (PTSD) in older females. She puts forth that sexual abuse and domestic physical violence renders women, and particularly older women, at heightened risk for PTSD –especially misdiagnosed PTSD. Eating disorders among older women is addressed by Brandsma (in Malatesta, 2007). Countering the notion that eating disorders are more or less isolated to the young female sector, the researcher notes recent work that indicates its incidence throughout the lifecourse. In particular, middle-aged and older women may be susceptible to binge eating. Finally, we note that Brandsma hones in on adult developmental experiences that may precipitate an eating disorder in this group.

Mental Health among Female Children

In the United States, children's mental disorders are considered a serious public health issue. Based on the National Research Council and Institute of Medicine report (Preventing mental, emotional, and behavioral disorders among young people: Progress and possibilities, 2009) approximately 13 –20% of children living in America report a mental disorder in a given year, and the yearly health burden amounts to approximately $247 billion.
Globally, the mental health of female children is highly affected by myriad factors ranging from sexual abuse and trafficking to female infanticide, FGM/C and early/forced marriage. These topics will be explored in their wider context in subsequent sections of this chapter, and in the context of the Arab Middle East in the subsequent chapter.

Here, we select just several points. Spataro, Mullen, Burgess, Wells and Moss (2004) examined the impact of child sexual abuse on mental health. Their study (N=1612) was unusual in that it showed, prospectively, a definite link between child sexual abuse that was validated at the time the abuse occurred and serious mental illness in both childhood and adult life. At the same time, the study did not provide support for the frequently advanced notion of a relationship between child sexual abuse and psychosis.

Taking account of child abuse from a different perspective, Afifi and von Bothmer (2007) explored the associations between Egyptian women's attitudes on FGM/C and maternal child abuse. Specifically, they tested the link between physical abuse of their children in the month immediately preceding the investigation and their beliefs about FGM/C. We shall return to this paper in the section on FGM/C in the Arab region, but here we simply note that these authors found that holding positive beliefs about the practice of FGM/C or having the intention to continue the practice was linked with maternal physical abuse.

Mental Health Disorders among Women in Under-served Populations

Despite wide-ranging mental health needs among women globally, the focus on helping women in under-served populations has been quite narrow, mostly centering on family planning (WHO, 1993). Nonetheless, across cultures and regions, women in under-served populations are at a higher risk than men for affective disorders (Desjarlais, Eisenberg, Good & Kleinman 1995). In less-developed countries, nearly 30% of disability related to psychiatric illness among women was related to depression, as compared to only 12.6% among men (World Bank, 1993). However, fewer than half those affected by depression have access to the well-known treatments available (e.g., psychosocial support, cognitive behavioral therapies and anti-depression medication); in some countries, that number plummets to 10% (WHO, 2012). Despite the known effectiveness of treatment for depression, the majority of people in need do not receive it. Throughout the world, barriers to treatment include social stigma associated with emotional illness, as well as lack of funds and paucity of treatment professionals (Depression, A Global Crisis, 2012). Even in developed societies, stigma has been identified as a primary obstacle to mental health provision. Osman and Al-Radi (2005) note that the U.S. Surgeon General described stigma as 'the most formidable obstacle to future progress in the arena of mental illness and health' (p. 19).

A range of suggestions have been offered for the sex variance in rates of mental disorders (Paykel, 1991). These include gender differences in distress awareness and management, biological factors, and social determinants. The latter has been seen by some scholars as preeminent, with low SES (socio-economic status) and conflictual partner relationships major factors in emotional distress (Blue I, Ducci ME, & Jaswal S., 1995). In point of fact, the determinants of mental illness are quite interwoven. As an example, one may take what has been termed the 'feminization of poverty' (i.e., women constituting two-thirds of the 2.5 billion people living on less than US $2 per day) (DCAF, 2005). Poverty has been widely noted to be a major factor in women's vulnerability to violence. In other words, with no alternative means of support, women may remain with violent partners or sex-trafficking bosses (DCAF, 2005). We shall now outline several of these scenarios.

Violence against Women (VAW)

Violence against women (hereinafter, VAW) has garnered a great deal of academic and popular interest in the last several decades (Gill, 2009; Heise, Ellsberg & Gottemoeller, 1999; Heise, Pitanguy & Germain, 1994). Horvath & Kelly (2006) have noted the recent work on a range of VAW, including intimate partner violence, sexual violence, forced marriage and female genital mutilation (FGM). 'Honor' crimes, female infanticide, and 'dowry' killings/bride burnings constitute specific forms of VAW.

Women between the ages of fifteen and forty-four have a greater chance of being hurt or killed as a result of male violence than from cancer, traffic accidents, malaria and war combined (DCAF, 2005). Victims/survivors of VAW are at increased risk for a range of adverse emotional, physical and reproductive outcomes (Al-Nsour, Khawaja & Al-Kayyali, 2009).

Intimate Partner Violence (IPV)

The scope of the problem of intimate partner violence toward women is extraordinarily extensive. Indeed, among a range of VAW, intimate partner violence was ranked highest (Faramarzi, Esmailzadeh, & Mosavi, 2005). The median prevalence of IPV worldwide is 21% (Al-Nsour et al., 2009), with the prevalence in developing countries estimated between 18-67% (Al-Nsour et al., 2009). Unsurprisingly, women who have been abused experience significantly higher rates of emotional distress, as compared to non-abused women (Al-Nsour et al., 2009). Battered women commonly report a range of complaints, including depression, post-traumatic stress disorder, anxiety, alcohol use disorders, and somatic symptoms (Al-Nsour et al., 2009).

The prevalence of violence against women in the United States is very high. According to the US Department of Health and Human Services, Centers for Disease Control:

> Violence against women is a substantial public health problem in the United States. According to data from the criminal justice system, hospital and medical records, mental health records, social services, and surveys, thousands of women are injured or killed each year as a result of violence, many by someone they are involved with or were involved with intimately. Nearly one-third of female homicide victims reported in police records are killed by an intimate partner (Federal Bureau of Investigation 2001, cited in CDC, 2003, p. 2).

Specifically:

> The costs of intimate partner rape, physical assault, and stalking exceed $5.8 billion each year, nearly $4.1 billion of which is for direct medical and mental health care services. The total costs of IPV also include nearly $0.9 billion in lost productivity from paid work and household chores for victims of nonfatal IPV and $0.9 billion in lifetime earnings lost by victims of IPV homicide (CDC, 2003, p. 1).

Moving to the situation in less-developed regions, a 2005 WHO study on domestic violence against women in 10 mainly developing countries found that 'among women aged 15-49, between 15% of women in Japan and 71% of women in Ethiopia reported violence at the hands of an intimate partner in their lifetime; between 0.3–11.5% of women reported experiencing sexual violence by a non-partner since the age of 15 years; the first sexual experience for many women was reported as forced – 17% in rural Tanzania, 24% in rural Peru, and 30% in rural Bangladesh' (p.3). The bulk of this violence is IPV. Nearly one-third of all women globally who have been in a partner-relationships have experienced violence at the hands of their intimate partner, and in some areas the numbers rise precipitously. Up to 38% of all murders of women are committed by intimate partners (WHO, 2013).

Men are typically the perpetrators in IPV and sexual violence; women are typically the victims. Depression, post-traumatic stress disorder, sleep disorders, substance disorders and suicide attempts on the part of the victim are associated with intimate partner violence. Women who have experienced intimate partner violence are almost twice as likely as non-abused women to report depression and alcohol-use disorders. For those who were the victims of non-partner sexual violence, the rate was even higher (WHO, 2013).

Dowry Death'/'Bride Burning'

'Dowry Death' is a term for a type of VAW in which a woman is killed in ostensible retaliation for her family's reneging on dowry-related promises – or their inability to fulfill demands that have been increased since the wedding. Because immolation is frequently the means of murder, the term 'bride burning' is also used in the literature for this crime (Heise et al., 1994). Dowry death (or bride burning) takes place throughout the world, but occurs most frequently in South Asia. The victim's husband or parents-in-law are typically the perpetrators (Heise et al., 1994 and Desjarlais et al., 1995). According to the Indian National Crime Records Bureau, 8,233 Indian women were killed in 2012 in dowry-related violence, and the incidence of dowry killings grew by nearly 3% over the previous five years (*The Times of India*, 2013). However, as rates of reporting this crime are considered to be low, the statistics may not reflect its actual prevalence.

Journalist Nalini Singh maintains that 'dowry-death' is a misnomer in that this crime only *appears* to be dowry-driven. In reality, she writes, the 'dowry death' itself is typically the culmination of a personal history of emotional and physical assault toward the victim perpetrated by her husband and/or his parents. This violence, she claims, is part and parcel of a patriarchal stance of lack of female worth (*PUCL Bulletin*, 1982). Thus, while there are few survivors of dowry-related crimes, women in South Asia are at risk for the wide-ranging emotional and physical distress associated with this violent outcome. Further, dowry-related problems may impact on many aspects of a woman's life, such as considerations of bearing and raising a female child (see below).

Female Infanticide

Anthropologist Laila Williamson contends that infanticide has been practiced for centuries across regions and cultures. In fact, Williamson conceived of it as the rule rather than the exception (Milner, 2000). Larry S. Milner, a physician and infanticide researcher, reckons that it was only the relative availability of safe and legal means of abortion that has largely shifted the contemporary western perspective on infanticide: where available, it has eased the perceived need to kill an infant after its birth. In his work on the history of infanticide, Milner notes that, historically, poverty seems to have driven parents (often the mother) to kill her newborn child, especially if it was a girl – a girl, after, all, was subject to dowry demands and would traditionally transfer her earning power and physical support to her husband's family (Milner, 2000).

In the view of 1998 Nobel Laureate Amartya Sen, sex-selective abortions and female infanticide in North Africa, China, and South Asia account for the approximately six million 'demographically missing' women worldwide (DCAF, 2005). In one survey, more than half the women who were sampled in China reported that they had killed a baby daughter (Desjarlais et al., 1995). China's 'One child per family' governmental policy was intended to alleviate existing conditions of poverty, but exacerbated the pressure to produce a male child. Female-child neglect is not difficult to observe in China. The World Health Organization noted that mothers were more likely to seek medical care for their male children than their female children, the latter of whom may be typically treated at a later stage of disease than boys (Farah in *Gendercide Watch*, 1999-2013). Hence, in 2000, according to a Chinese census, the ratio of new-born girls to boys was 100:119, while the expected ratio was 100:103 (DCAF, 2005).

India, too, is considered a very bad place to be a female child. In 2012, the UN Department of Economic and Social Affairs reported that an Indian female between the ages of 1 -5 was 75% more likely to die than a boy her age (cited in Krishnan, 2012). Twelve million girls are born per year in India: one million of them die by their first birthdays (cited in Krishnan, 2012). Indian physician Anoop Saxena noted that while fetal sex determination is unlawful in India, it is widely practiced (DW, 2012). Thus, echoing Milner above, sex-selective abortion may be used in the service of privileging male children. Also in line with Milner, Gendercide Watch (1999-2013) states that infanticide is overwhelmingly perpetrated by the baby's mother.

Not only poverty, however, fuels female infanticide/sex-selective abortion. These acts have been noted to take place in India and China across socioeconomic fields. Reflective of this point, Sunita Kishor writes that in India, despite widespread gains in basic resources for subsistence, girls lag behind boys in likelihood of survival. In fact, agricultural development *decreases* the survival rate of females (males' survival rates are unaffected). Reminiscent of many scholars' opinions on patriarchal preferences for males in multiple arenas, the author attributes this fact to recalcitrant sex-based discrimination in the allocation of resources (Kishor, 2005).

Sexual Violence: Rape and Female Trafficking

Women are raped throughout the world, and particularly in regions experiencing social disintegration. According to the World Health Organization, approximately one woman in five will be the victim of rape or attempted rape in her lifetime (WHO, 2000). This ratio is one in six in Canada, New Zealand, the United Kingdom and the United States (UNDP, Human Development Report 1995 Gender and Human Development, p. 7). Rape of female minors is at epidemic proportions in some regions: forty percent of girls aged 17 or under in South Africa were the victim of rape or attempted rape (UN Habitat, State of the World's Cities: Trends in Sub-Saharan Africa: 2006).

In their work on the impact of rape, Morrison, (2007) described what they call the 'ripple effects' of this violence, highlighting the multiple costs of the perpetration on the victim's social network and the broader community as a whole. Psychological consequences of rape include fear of death and disassociation during the assault; anxiety and ongoing fears; poor self-esteem, self-blame, and guilt; shock, confusion, and denial; self-harm, suicidal ideation and attempted suicide and post-traumatic stress disorder (PTSD) (Morrison, 2007). Physical consequences of sexual assault may include chronic diseases, headaches, eating disorders, gynecological distress, irritable bowel syndrome, and damage to the genital area (Morrison, 2007). Intimate, friend and familial relationships may be affected by the sexual assault, and a victim's professional, social and communal life may change. 'Secondary victimization' may occur in conjunction with the victim's response to the criminal justice system and health service providers and in response to the reactions of significant others. Sexual assault typically results in financial costs related to both earnings and earning capacity, medical and psychological treatment, as well as a host of 'invisible' costs. Finally, and as mentioned above, as some cultures link female virginity with personal and family honor, forced marriage to the rapist and murder at the hands of a family member are very real possibilities in many communities (see chapter three) (Morrison, 2007).

Female Trafficking

Human trafficking for purposes of sexual exploitation has grown exponentially since the European slave trade of the nineteenth century, with globalization making the trade in humans easier than ever to manage (Chung, 2006). On an international scale, the business of human trafficking yields approximately $9.5 billion dollars per year, and is a prime source of profit for organized crime. The appeal of this activity is enhanced by the fact that legal penalties for human trafficking for sexual purposes are light as compared to trafficking even illegal objects. A United Nations report estimates that 700,000 to 2,000,000 women and children are trafficked per year on a global basis (Chung, 2006).

The movement of human trafficking is typically in the direction of less-developed to more-developed countries (e.g., to the United States and the European Union). Approximately 50,000 women and children are trafficked to the United States each year (CIA Report, 1999, cited in Chung, 2006) and 120,000 to the European Union (Chung, 2006). The bulk of these persons (30,000) are from Southeast Asia; 10,000 originate in Latin America, 4,000 in Eastern Europe, and 1,000 in other regions (Chung, 2006).

Trafficking victims are typically both poor and poorly educated, and they are lured by fake offers of foreign employment. Once in a country in which they do not speak the language, the identification papers of victims are taken away and they are forced into prostitution, told that they must pay off non-existent debt (Chung, 2006).

Some traditional cultural values render girls particularly vulnerable to trafficking. An example would be the Asian cultural value of filial obligation to parents, conjoined with general patriarchal views of women as less worthy than men – and in some cases, 'goods' to be marketed (see chapter one of this volume). As in other regions of the world, rape and prostitution carry a cultural stigma in Asia, resulting in familial shame. Return may be impossible for victims whose families have cut them off. (Chung, 2006)

Victims of human trafficking are frequently bought and sold repeatedly. Drugs and the threat of violence may be used to compel compliance. Seventy to 95% of sex workers report physical assault, 60% to 75% of prostitutes have been raped, and 89% of these persons wish to escape prostitution (Chung, 2006). Sexually transmitted diseases, including HIV/AIDS are a constant risk, as are pelvic diseases, forced substance abuse, damage to reproductive and other organs, unwanted pregnancy, forced abortion, and abortion-related complications. In addition, scabies, tuberculosis and hepatitis are among the communicable diseases that forever loom. Some scholars suggest a positive relationship between sex trafficking and the transmission of AIDs (Chung, 2006).

Concomitant with the physical are the emotional ramifications of human trafficking. These include helplessness and hopelessness, low self-esteem, self-blame, frank depression, anxiety, guilt, anger, rage, sleep disorders, loss of appetite and energy and suicidal ideation. The clinical criteria of post-traumatic stress disorder is met by 68% of persons who have been trafficked (Chung, 2006).

'Honor' Crimes against Women

Worldwide, approximately 5,000 women per year are killed in the name of 'honor crimes' (United Nations Population Fund UNFPA, cited in DCAF, 2005). Nadya Khalife, a researcher on women's rights in the Arab world for Human Rights Watch, affirms that 'honor crimes' occur in a number of locales: the Middle East, Pakistan, Bangladesh and among immigrant communities in North America. Several Arab countries and territories, including Iraq, Kuwait, Syria, Yemen and the Palestinian Authority-controlled territories of Israel, have laws providing lesser sentences for so-called 'honor' murders than for other murders (Human Rights Watch).

Egypt and Jordan also have laws that have been interpreted to allow reduced sentences for 'honor' crimes, according to Human Rights Watch. A study of female deaths in Egypt revealed that 47% of the victims were killed by a relative after the woman had been raped. Sometimes, the assault – perhaps with acid or fire - will leave the victim horribly disfigured, but alive.

'Honor' murders are a specific form of VAW. Scholars debate the independence of the crime from the category of general domestic violence, as well as the relationship it might (or might not) have with religion (see chapter three). We will return to this topic in the next chapter.

For now, we will consider the phenomenon of 'honor killings' in the United States. According to Farhana Qazi, a Lecturer on Muslim conflicts, while the prevalence of act in America is very low, the country is by no means immune to the scourge:

In Islam, a girl has a right to choose her spouse. She has a right to fall in love. And she even has a right to file for divorce. Numerous examples in Islamic history prove women are free agents, not subservient actors. But honor killings discredit Islam and reflect a more powerful cultural value. The men who kill (or dictate in) the name of honor decide the roles of their women and their fate, even in America (*The Islamic Monthly*, 2014, online).

Mei Mei Fox (*The Huffington Post*, September 16, 2014) reported on a new documentary titled *The Price of Honor*, treating the subject of 'honor killing.' The movie open with an audio recording of an emergency call placed by Texas teenager Sarah Said screaming that her father is shooting her and her elder sister Amina. The two sisters were killed that day, on January 1, 2008. The murderer, their father, Yaser Said, stated that he was 'defending the family honor.'

The United States is beginning to respond. According to Fox, the U.S. Department of Justice is investigating how best to gather information on honor violence in America: the target goal for strategy development was early 2015. Further, the U.S. State Department now categorizes forced GM/C and forced marriage as forms of honor violence, and has established task forces for both issues. In America, forced marriage (which was being imposed on Amina Said) is currently prohibited in only nine states. At this point, we shall discuss briefly these practices from a global perspective.

Female Genital Mutilation/Cutting (FGM/C)

The World Health Organization (2014) writes that FGM/C refers to all procedures that involve the partial or total removal of the external female genitalia, or other injury to the female genital organs for non-medical purposes. WHO further notes that FGM/C:

> (1)' has no health benefits for girls and women', (2) 'can cause severe bleeding and problems urinating, and later cysts, infections, infertility as well as complications in childbirth and increased risk of newborn deaths'; that 'more than 125 million girls and women alive today have been cut in the 29 countries in Africa and the Middle East where FGM is concentrated' and that FGM is mostly carried out on young girls sometime between infancy and age 15 (WHO, 2014, p. 1).

Razor blades, glass, kitchen knives, scissors, and human teeth are some of the implements that have been used in the procedure (Council on Scientific Affairs, AMA, 1995, p.. 1714; cited in Al-Krenawi and Wiesel-Lev, 1999). Some improvements have been made in recent years, increasing the rates of sterility of FGM/C (Elgousi, 2013), but conditions in rural and remote areas continue to be extremely dangerous. Even when medical professionals are involved, the current situation endangers the lives of young women. We shall learn in the next chapter of one such example, but here we will take note of the research of Cathleen M. Braddy and Julia A. Files, who studied clinical considerations related to FGM/C cases in the United States. Addressing the increasing prevalence of the practice among US residents, these researchers write that, 'An understanding of the short- and long-term complications of FGM is also essential, because US clinicians are increasingly encountering girls and women who have had FGM' (Braddy & Files, 2007, p. 162).

Here too, scholars debate the association between this set of procedures and religion, and we will explore the physical and mental health consequences in chapter four.

Early/Forced Marriage

Although early/forced marriage is particularly prevalent in Africa and Asia, it is a world-wide problem (United Nations Human Rights Office, 2013). Globally, one out of seven girls is married before she turns 15, and some are married by the age eight. They may be married to any male, of any age, and their early marriage puts them at an enhanced risk of injury or death from childbirth, poverty, HIV/ AIDS and intimate partner violence (UN Human Rights Office, 2013).

Having considered women's mental health from a wider-angle lens of the global frame, we now narrow the aperture and view the topic from the vantage point of Arab/Muslim women in the Arab Middle East.

Chapter 4
Women's Mental Health in the Middle East

Overview

As discussed in the previous chapter, women throughout the world are challenged by an impressive host of social, cultural, economic and biological factors in the maintenance of their mental health. In this chapter, we zero in on the mental health of women in the Middle East, examining how women in this region fare with regard to emotional distress, particularly in light of the specific cultural conditions found in the MENA region. In the first section, we will review the most salient categories explored earlier, noting the variations for Arab women as compared to their western counterparts regarding depression, anxiety disorders and somatization behavior. As well, we will note issues of comorbidity that have been found in the Arab region. Next, we will discuss a number of culture-specific points pertaining to the ways in which Middle Eastern persons construct notions of honor, both personal and familial – although, as we will see, in this context these topics are highly imbricated. In the final section, we will explore some particular ways in which the interpenetration of culture and religion in the Arab region serves to erect major obstacles to mental health for women in the Middle East: these include the acceptance and even promotion of 'honor' crimes, early/forced marriage, polygyny and FGM.

We begin with Josi Agnes Salem-Pickartz, who underscores the nascent quality of the inquiry into mental health concerns currently taking place in the Middle East:

> Mental health (Arabic, *al-siḥḥa al-nafsiyya*) is a social construct whose meaning varies across the scientific, social, and religious communities in the Arab countries. A gendered understanding of mental health is, however, in its very beginnings (Salem-Pickartz, 2015).

In the previous chapter, we touched upon the fact that, across the globe, the investigation of women's health in general and women's mental health in particular is in its infancy. In this chapter, we go further, and note that in a region only beginning to take up the call for a broad research perspective on mental health, the body of knowledge on Arab women's mental health is currently in skeletal form.

Depression

While depression ranks extremely high in mental health burden the world over, particularly for women, the prevalence of depression among women in the Middle East constitutes an amplified cause for concern. Recent data from the Institute for Health Metrics and Evaluations (IHME) indicates that women in this region are more prone to depression than women anywhere else on the globe. While the Arab world's men were also found to have an enhanced risk of depression relative to the male world population, the gap between males and females was greater than elsewhere, excepting Latin America and the Caribbean. Thus, the prevalence of depression among men in the Middle East is in relative accord with their counterparts across the globe – unlike depression among women in this region, which exceeds the already high global rate (Freund, 2013).

Awareness of this phenomenon is growing. A 2012 medical conference in Dubai was dedicated to the issue of depression among women in the MENA region, and a second such conference is scheduled for March, 2015. Psychologist Saliha Afridi highlighted at the congress the stigma experienced by Arab women who seek western mental health care. Afridi noted that in the Arab region, disclosure of familial dysfunction to outsiders remains anathema. This echoes Al-Krenawi et al. (2000), who found that 'women in Arab society are profoundly reluctant to seek mental health treatment' (cited in Al-Krenawi & Graham, 2004, p. 141). Chaleby and Racy (1999) explained the under-representation of women in psychiatric hospital data to vigorous efforts on the part of the patient's family to conceal information on emotional distress so as to safeguard marital prospects. This longstanding stigma has been noted in multiple investigations of psycho-social interventions among ethnic Arabs. Not only are future marital possibilities at issue, but the need for psychological treatment may be leveraged by the husband or his family of origin for entering into polygyny (Al-Krenawi, 1998a; Al-Krenawi et al., 1997). In the view of Salem-Pickartz (2015), women in Arab cultures take tremendous pains to avoid being labeling as 'al-junun'; that is, crazy. The social repercussions for female emotional disorder in the Arab world are fierce. As one scholar put it, 'A crazy woman [in the Arab region] is usually excluded from her social contacts and is controlled, confined, and often punished by her family' (Salem-Pickartz, p. 270). In chapter seven we shall delve into the concept of 'al-junun.'

Thus, rather than women directly seeking mental health support, primary care physicians typically wind up hearing the psychosomatic reports of emotionally distressed women (Afridi, 2012, Al-Krenawi, 2004).The recent conference devoted to depression among women in Arab regions, then, clearly mirrors the findings on somatization behavior in primary care settings discussed in chapter 3, once more paralleling but sometimes surpassing the level of psychological distress in more western, less traditional communities.

Hamdan, Hawamdeh, and Hussein (2008) found that depressive symptoms are common among women in primary health care centers in the Emirate of Sharjah. Significantly, these authors further noted that research on mental health needs of women in the Arab region is still in its infancy, and urge Arab states to actively and vigorously consider the social, psychological, and economic variables that impact on emotional health in the Middle East. In the context of Turkey, Tuncer (in Al-Issa, 1995) noted being that female was one of several risk factors for depression.

Transcultural Issues in Differential Diagnosis

Somatization

The issue of differential diagnosis of depression in the Arab world was taken up by Amin, Hamdi and Abou-Saleh (cited in Okasha & Maj, 2001). They address what they term the 'national identity' of depression as it presents in ethnic Arab persons (p. 90). Notable are the standardized instruments used in the study of depression: El-Islam et al. (1988), in using a western-derived instrument, the Standardized Assessment of Depressive Disorders, needed in their work among Kuwaitis to add a category in order to cover phenomena that were not included in the protocol. Hamdi, Amin and Abou-Saleh (1997) noted that depression among Arab patients may present with behavior not usually associated with the disorder. Amin et al. (2001) point out that both the main western diagnostic manuals (DSM of the American Psychiatric Association and the ICD-10) offer some flexibility in presentations of depression, and, further, that, 'In Arab patients, these variations are quite significantly present and characteristic' (p. 98). Specifically, they cite a great deal of work in which somatization behaviors figure prominently in depression in Arab patients (Tuncer, 1995; El-Islam et al., 1988; Karam et al., 1998; El-Islam, 1969; Abou-Saleh, 1994).

Postpartum Depression

Postpartum depression in the region has received some scholarly attention. An early study in the field for the MENA region, Ghoubash and Abou-Saleh (1997) found that the 95 postpartum women they sampled in the UAE reported rates of depression in line with those reported in the West. More recently, Bener, Burgut, Ghuloum, and Sheikh (2011) studied postpartum depression in what they refer to as a 'fast-developing country' (Qatar). With a primary care center as the research venue and a large sample size (N=1379), these researchers they also wrote of a prevalence comparable to that reported in previous epidemiological studies conducted in developed societies. Like Ghubash and Abou-Saleh as well as many other scholars, Bener et al. (2011) stressed the urgent need for constructing a knowledge base on women's depression in this region. In this direction, Glasser, Tanous, Shihab, Ziv, Goldman, and Kaplan (2011). noted that the rate of pre- and postnatal depression among Arab women in northern Israel was slightly higher than that of Jewish Israeli women living in the same area, and quite a bit lower than that of Arab Bedouin women in southern Israel. Indeed, the latter population was found by Glasser (2011) to have a strikingly high rate of postpartum depression, relative to their Israeli Jewish counterparts. Following Bener et al. (2011), we might call the Arab Bedouin communities 'fast-developing'; this rate of postpartum depression may be reflective of the special circumstances in which they live, as noted in chapter six.

Anxiety

The prevalence of anxiety disorders among Arab women in the Middle East is comparable to that of women throughout the world (Hamdan, 2009). Karam et al. (2006) showed in a large-sample epidemiological study in Lebanon, that the 12-month prevalence of anxiety disorders was

11.2%, in line with results in developed countries. Being female was found to be associated with mood and anxiety disorders (Hamdan, 2009). In a large-scale study across 10 Arab countries, Abdel-Khalek (2004) studied sex differences in anxiety among university undergraduates. The Kuwait University Anxiety Scale (KUAS) was used in its Arabic form. Across countries, female participants were found to have higher mean anxiety scores than did male participants. Kardi et al. (2007) studied 800 participants in Morocco, and found that 25.5% met the criteria for at least one anxiety disorder. Women constituted the 'overwhelming majority' of cases for the following anxiety disorders: social phobia, obsessive-compulsive disorder, generalized anxiety disorder, panic disorder and PTSD (cited in Hamdan, 2009, p. 596).

Somatization Behaviors

Researchers have found a high prevalence of somatization behaviors among ethnic Arabs (Dwairy, 1998). Becker (2004) studied somatization behavior in Saudi Arabia, and found a 19% prevalence rate; fully 70% of this group was female (cited in Hamdan, 2009). Especially significant in light of the high rates of depression now being recognized among women in the Arab region (see above) some researchers maintain that somatization behavior among ethnic Arab patients particularly, masks depression and anxiety (El-Islam, 1995). Along these lines, in their work with Bedouin Arab women in southern Israel Al-Krenawi & Graham (2004) found high rates of somatization behavior. This behavior was especially pronounced among divorced Arab women, which they argue is reflective of the unmet psychosocial needs of Arab women in general in patriarchal cultures. These needs have been noted to be related to consequences of divorce for women in the Arab culture (Brhoom, 1987; cited in Al-Krenawi & Graham, 2004; El-Saadani, 2006). This point will be taken up in greater depth in chapter eight of this volume.

Comorbidity in the MENA region

Recent years have witnessed some ground-breaking work on the comorbidity of depression with chronic diseases among Arab persons in the MENA region. For instance, Elshahawi, Hussein, Mobarak and Enas

(2011) investigated depression comorbidity among patients with chronic hepatitis C (HCV). A cross-sectional, controlled study was carried out in Egypt on 200 subjects with CHC. The authors concluded that depression is quite prevalent in patients with CHC; the depression was much more severe among those on interferon therapy as compared to those not receiving interferon.

Kilzieh et al. (2008) set out to examine the comorbidity of chronic illness and depression in Aleppo, Syria. The researchers performed a cross-sectional, population-based study on Syrian adults (N=2038) using a structured interview questionnaire. Kilzieh and colleagues concluded that in the Aleppo community, depression is linked with multiple chronic disorders which include: chronic respiratory diseases, hypertension, peptic ulcer disease and kidney disease. Moreover, the authors identified an important gender-related risk factor: the results of an association between depression and SES (socio-economic status) held only among the female subjects. The results, then, confirm 'the recurrent finding of women's higher vulnerability to the adverse mental health effects of lower SES' (Kilzieh et al., 2008, p. 179).

In a related inquiry, Kilzieh et al. (2010) sought to investigate associations between physical impairment, gender, depression and SES in Aleppo, Syria. In this first epidemiological study of physical impairment in Syria, impairment was found to be significantly associated with being a woman and having a low SES. Notably, these results shed light on a major topic of the current volume: the multifarious ramifications of gender disparity in the Arab world. Citing Ballantyne (1999), who proposed that the effect of poor SES on health is mediated by gender, thus resulting in compromised health among women, the authors suggest that low SES, and not depression or chronic diseases, mostly explained the above-noted finding. Second, and again in line with research on this topic done in the West (e.g., Bruffaerts & Ormel, 2006; Hays, Wells, Sherbourne, Rogers & Spritzer, 1995; Wells, Golding & Burnam, 1988), this study found that physical impairment too was associated with depression. The authors suggest that the latter finding may be mediated through co-existing chronic diseases. In a final and critical point, the researchers note the 'prominent stigma' associated with the diagnosis and treatment of psychological disorders in Syria, which they believe is likely to result in under-diagnosis of depression. Below, we engage with this topic.

Constructions of stigma in the Arab region

El-Islam (1998, cited in El-Islam, 2008) writes of the prevalence of 'associated stigma,' in Islamic culture; that is, shame that is experienced by the family of an individual who is behaving in a way that is considered as 'abnormal' (p. 674). The stigma of mental illness is related to this code of collectivist honor. An individual who is too sick to be responsible for keeping his or her own behavior within the confines of cultural norms has lost his or her dignity. This concerns the emotionally ill person, and it is equally if not more true of the individual who has 'lost' her sexual dignity (and by extension, the dignity of her family).

As noted above, stigma pertaining to disclosure of Arab persons' emotional distress has been thought to go hand-in-hand with the underdiagnosing of depression in this region, and, especially, to an underreporting of psychological problems among Arab women (Afridi, 2012). Researchers have contended, as well, that the latter group's emotional distress is typically de-legitimized in the MENA region (Abu-Baker, 2005). Dwairy (1998) too writes that Arab women may have an enhanced likelihood of being affected by stigma around psychological distress. In their work on reduction of stigma pertaining to mental illness in the Middle East, Sewilam et al. (2014) note that stigma around this issue has indeed persisted in the region. These authors write of a number of ways in which Arab persons in emotional distress attempt to reduce the associated burden of stigma. These include 'somatization' of the distress (Okasha & Karam, 1998) echoing the beginning of this chapter and research indeed found throughout this book; and recourse to a faith healer (Okasha & Karam, 1998). Further supporting the interrelatedness of salient social constructs, Al-Issa (1995) speculates that the prevalence of somatization throughout the Arab region might be related to the diagnosing clinician's interest in helping the patient avoid the stigma of mental illness, a stigma, as described above, that permeates and informs daily life and has critical ramifications for Arab persons. This may be especially true for Arab women, as we will see below.

While there is limited research on coterminous traditional and biomedical treatment, this is becoming a topic of urgent interest in current world health strategies (see, for example, WHO, Traditional Medicine Strategy, 2014-2013) and notable exceptions exist. Below, we will explore an early case in which an initial western diagnosis was augmented by traditional intervention, resulting in the cessation of 'paranoid' symptomology and the restoration of family equilibrium that had been marred by suspicions concerning family 'honor.'

Female Subordination in the Middle East and its Effects on Mental Health

Belief systems are composite entities, interweaving thought systems, cultural creations and temporal needs. And so it is no surprise that El-Islam (in Okasha and Maj, 2001) asserts that belief systems in the Arab world are multi-determined. In the case of the Arab region, they stem from both Islamic and non-Islamic sources. The author cites the longstanding subordinate status of women in the region as a pre-Islamic posture that held fast even after the advent of Islam. Putting it sharply, one scholar of Islam has written that, 'Islam is the home of the eternal masculine' (Berque, 1964, cited in Racy, 1980, p. 213).

Time has not made the inroads for which one might have hoped. This persistent inferior social standing was highlighted very recently by Douki, et al. (2007) when they reported starkly that, 'Being a woman is still a misfortune in the Muslim world' (p. 180). These researchers attribute this situation to an overriding patriarchal perspective, as well as the strong cultural notion that women have the potential to sully the 'family honor' (see below). Further revealing the traditional Arab attitude toward female children, El-Islam (in Al-Issa, 2000) wrote that in its negativity it is '...only surpassed... by the [traditional] Chinese, who have a saying: It is better to raise geese than daughters' (p. 123; Tseng and McDermot, 1981). While in chapter four we discussed the 'missing' females in global demographic terms, spotlighting India and China, in this section we discuss the 'missing' females in the Arab region, that is, those who face not only gender inequality, but gender-driven mental and physical health problems which are tightly bound to a range of Islamic/Arabic cultural beliefs and behaviors. El-Islam (2001) has stated unequivocally that 'cultural factors, arising mainly from the subordinated position of women in Arab communities influence the prevalence, pattern and management of psychiatric disorders in women' (cited in Douki, et al. 2007, p. 179).

Porous Family Boundaries: Advantages and Disadvantages

The emotional, social and economic advantages of the high-context, low-individuation traditional Arab family/community have been quite well documented (Hall, 1976; Dwairy, 1998; Al-Krenawi, 2014; El-Islam, 2012;

Abu-Baker, 2005, Joseph, 1996). Powerfully, the Arab tradition of caring for challenged individuals encompasses the notion of *right*; that is, in the Arab world, it is both a right and a responsibility to care for less-advantaged members of society (Dwairy, 1998). Thus, the sense of privilege combines with the sense of obligation in performing this sort of difficult act. The traditional community essentially absorbs those with mild retardation, for instance, providing them with skill-appropriate tasks rather than institutionalizing them. The return-to-family-support agenda developed out of necessity by mental health systems in the West that have run out of money and living quarters for those with chronic psychiatric illnesses provides pause for the wholesale rejection of traditional management of illness (El-Islam in Okasha & Maj, 2001). El-Islam (2008) has proposed that the traditional Arab family may be well suited to serve as caregiver for those with emotional illness, even capable of devising particular individualized programs of support for psychiatrically distressed family members. Further, this type of extended family is well-positioned 'to provide a structure for their members that may sometimes prevent and or compensate for the effects of parental loss and mental disability' (p. 671). In short, the traditional Arab family, as compared to the typical western nuclear family, is by its nature built to be a safety net for its weakest members.

Nonetheless, the fluidity that marks the bounds of the self, so characteristic of the Arab family (see Joseph, chapter one of this volume), has been shown to be dual-edged. Ethnic Arab families in the Middle East tend to negatively assess emotional distress (Okasha, 2012) and may deem psychological illness to be a familial disgrace (Dwairy, 1998). This sensitivity to family honor extends well beyond mental illness, and encompasses all manner of sexual, and especially female sexual, behavior. Thus, the hypothetical safety net provided by the tight-knit Arab family may fail when female members, especially, are considered to have put into question the moral standing of the family. We will now explore the concept family honor, an issue that fraught with cultural meaning in the Arab tradition. We will see that while women as well as men participate in its social construction, it takes a direct toll on women's mental (and physical) health.

Constructions of Honor in the Arab Region

Two types of 'honor' are traditionally delineated in Arab society. The first is conveyed by the Arabic term *'ard,'* which may be translated roughly as 'chastity.' While by Islamic law both sexes are expected to uphold strict norms of sexual modesty and propriety, it is Arab/Islamic women who in a practical way are held to a very high standard in this regard (Abu-Rabia Queder, 2007). Thus, this form of honor pertains specifically to a woman's sexual demeanor and conduct. The term, which has deep roots in Arab society (Al-Krenawi, 2014), is highly related to another term, *'sharaf,'* which refers to the honor of a social unit, such as a family or a tribe (Feldner, 2000), together, these concepts constitute a great deal of cultural capital in the Arab/Islamic world.

As set out in chapter one, Arab culture is powerfully collectivistic. Family members trade security for conformity to the cultural code (El-Islam in Al-Issa, 2000). However, the ramifications of breaking the rules are grim. In the view of one scholar:

> Under the Arab code of honor, Muslims are taught to abdicate our individuality and accept our fate as the property of our families. Our lives don't belong to us; our lives belong to our tribes...if you cross their moral boundaries, you 'dishonor' many more beside yourself (Manji, 2011, Kindle edition, no pagination).

The repercussions for 'dishonor[ing] many more beside yourself' is the subject of the next sections in this chapter.

'Honor-Based' Violence in the Arab Region

In the past decade, research attention has begun to be trained on the issue of violence against women in Arab societies (Ennaji and Sadiqui, 2011; Chaudhry, 2013; Salhi, 2010). Zahia Smail Salhi has noted that:

> In MENA as in other regions in the world, culture is often violently masculinized, so that particular countries or nation-states are marked by their crimes against women. As such, Egypt and Sudan are characterized by female genital mutilation, Lebanon and other countries are known for honour killings (Salhi, 2010, p. 2).

As a working definition of honor-based violence, Aisha Gill (2009) suggests:

> ...violehnce perpetrated against females within the framework of patriarchal family structures, communities, and/or societies, where the main justification

for the perpetration of violence is the protection of a social construction of honor as a value system, norm, or tradition' (Gill, 2009, p.3).

The most extreme example of honor-based violence, honor-based murder, involves the murder, or attempted murder, of a woman by members of her family who do not approve of her sexual behavior (Abu-Odeh, 1996; Werbner, 2007, cited in Gill, 2009).

We saw in the previous chapter that VAW is ubiquitous, leaving no place on earth free of its mark. Especially pronounced, however, in the Arab/ Islamic region, is the communal perception of VAW, and 'honor-based' VAW in particular. Yotam Feldner (2000) stressed that in Arab culture, the salvaging of family 'honor' by murder of women perceived to be intimate with a (non-spousal) male is promoted by the family, village and tribal group. Investigating the confessions of such killers, he determined that the murder is typically encouraged by extended family and the wider social group. Thus, in the Arab world 'honor-based' violence against women, including 'honor' killings, are is not perpetrated by an individual, reacted to with abhorrence by the greater community. To the contrary, as we will see below, it can be part and parcel of the community ethos.

Further, these sentiments are not isolated to older individuals. A recent investigation of honor-based attitudes among teenagers in Jordan, for instance, found that one-third of respondents agreed with the practice of honor killing (Eisner & Ghuneim, 2013). Poor education and a patriarchal perspective, the latter working in conjunction with a preoccupation with female sexual virtue, were suggested by the researchers to be the core of the problem. Nonetheless:

> While we found the main demographic in support of HKA (honor killing attitudes) to be boys in traditional families with low levels of education, we noted substantial minorities of girls, well-educated and even irreligious teenagers who consider honor killing morally right, suggesting a persisting society-wide support for the tradition (Cambridge University News, 20 June 2013, no pagination).

This inquiry into youthful attitudes toward 'honor-based' violence has echoes in the work of Obeid, Chang and Ginges (2010) presented later in the chapter. These researchers investigated beliefs about wife beating among Lebanese students, and determined, among other points, that the respondents evinced a marked sympathy for wife battery following adulterous behavior of the wife.

Along the lines of Eisner's evaluation of the 'persisting society-wide support for the tradition [of 'honor killing'], it is becoming clear that public exposure of crimes such as these entails running up against a wall of taboo. In the context of Palestinian enclaves within Israel, Palestinian journalist Naela Khalil notes, 'Here, the family is stronger than even the security forces. I might criticise [Palestinian Authority President] Mahmoud Abbas more easily than a father or a brother who killed a woman. Doing this may mean a struggle with a whole family or village' (Breaking Israel News, 2013).

Thus, 'honor-based' violence against women is notoriously difficult to pin down and prosecute. Phyllis Chesler (2009) writes pointedly that as the motivation for 'honor' killing is to redeem purportedly besmirched family honor, families involved in the crime shy away from research and media attention, as those would bring precisely the opposite of the intended goal. 'Going missing' and claiming suicide are typical explanations for the sudden disappearance of the victim. Nonetheless, progressively, honor crimes are becoming more subject to investigation (Chesler, 2009). With respect to such investigations in the Middle East, Israel and Jordan provide two telling locales: each has been the focal point of recent academic and media interest.

In Israel, several instances of 'honor killings' have been brought to public light, thanks in part to the nearly unprecedented willingness of the families to speak with the media. In one case, a young, divorced Muslim Arab woman living in Deir al-Ghusun in the West Bank was murdered by her father, who was, according the victim's mother, under massive communal pressure to respond to a circulated petition (signed by a Palestinian lawmaker, among others) to 'reinstate the cultural and religious morals of his family.' In the view of the victim's mother, her husband simply cracked under the social pressure, and, against his true nature, committed the murder (*The Jerusalem Post*, 2013). This victim was the twenty-seventh one in a single year identified by police in Palestinian-run areas of Israel as murdered on the pretext of 'honor.'

In a second publicized case, forced marriage was the precipitating event. According to the seventeen year-old Muslim victim's mother, the daughter was killed by her brothers for rejecting an arranged marriage plan with a cousin who wished to marry her. The mother of the victim spoke to the authorities after this latest of multiple-per-year 'honor murders' in the West Bank town of Ramallah (Pelham, 2014).

The cases in Jordan share many elements with those in Israel. First, reduced penalties for men committing so-called honor crimes are common to both Palestinian Authority regions in the West Bank and to Jordan. According to a 2007 UN analysis, the Jordanian penal code is lenient with those who invoke the principle of family honor when committing violent crimes, including murder, against women. 'Premeditated murder in Jordan is punishable by death, but the penal code exempts from the death penalty men who kill female relatives found committing adultery. Instead, men committing honour crimes receive short prison sentences' (UN Report, 2007). Second, as in Palestinian-controlled areas in the West Bank, both culture and politics play pivotal roles in holding fast to the 'honor-violence' status quo. According to Reem Abu Hassan, an attorney and leading women's rights activist in Jordan:

> There is no political will to fight so-called honour crimes. The tribal mentality is the main driving force that makes this phenomenon spin out of control. We have to change the whole mentality of the nation (p.1).

Third, there is a similar, overarching cultural component. In an explanation that could have been describing 'honor' murders in Arab communities in Israel, Abu Hassan spoke of how communities view the perpetrators as the true victims, having been 'shamed' by their female relatives. From adolescent flirtation to full sexual relationships with men, familial disgrace is at stake in the sexual conduct of a family's female members. To illustrate, according to Asma Khader, Jordanian minister of state and government spokesperson, when 'honor' killers turn themselves in to the police, 'the police try to calm them down, give them a cigarette. The culture deals with them as heroes' (Human Rights Watch interview with Asma Khader, July 12, 2003). Fourth, in both areas, female as well as male family members have been complicit in the murders: mothers and sisters have assisted in the planning of such killings, and they have also murdered with their own hands.

The Jordanian case of Mohammad Rai deserves particular note, not for its singularity, but rather for the light it sheds on the complex of motivations inherent to the act of 'honor' killing. When Rai was 17 years old, he murdered his cousin 'to uphold his family's honour,' and 'he did it under pressure from family elders' (p. 1). In retrospect (and after having served a full sentence of six months in prison) Rai expressed no remorse; in fact, 'I would do it again if I had to. People here would have stigmatised my entire family if I had not killed her and shame would have followed us wherever we went.' Rai sums up: 'We are prisoners of our own social habits, there is nothing we can do about it.'

Rai's candid (if cold-blooded) review of his behavior reveals a number of important points. To begin with, Rai was a very young man, not out of his teens, when he murdered his cousin. An entire lifetime lay in front of him, and yet, exercising at least a certain level of volition (though he denies this, claiming to be a helpless 'prisoner of social habits') he killed his kin. According to Rai's account, he was vigorously deputized by older folks in the community to commit the murder. This line of conduct should be seen within its proper cultural context; that is, as El-Islam informs us (cited in Al-Issa, 2000, p. 123),'Respect for and obedience to elders top the list of family traditions…'). Protestations of helplessness aside, Rai might have been able to reject his assigned role, but in order to do so he likely would have had to escape from his entire social group: he would have had to leave his community – and possibly his country. There was no room for (at least public) dissent on this issue in Rai's sphere. On the contrary, there was unanimity on the inevitability of the murder ('People here would have stigmatized my entire family if I had not killed her.') Not just the elders, then, but everyone, it seems, expected this outcome. As a voluminous amount of research has proven (WHO, 2008), while VAW is globally prevalent, it is the societal expectation of this behavior in the Arab region that warrants particular note. Next, Rai's decision may have been colored by lenient Jordanian laws for this crime, as well as by expectations of the victim's family; his six-month-long prison stay was the result of the family of the victim dropping its charge. Finally, Rai offers the ultimate justification for the killing: '…shame would have followed us wherever we went.' While El-Islam (1982) refers to 'associative shame' in the context of mental health problems in the Arab world, perhaps it is reasonable to broaden its heuristic value and suggest that Rai, and others like him, experienced associative shame with regard to his cousin's alleged behavior. In fact, the prospect of familial shame transformed murder into proper behavior, necessary and correct given the circumstances.

Deepening the discussion, researchers Amalia Sa'ar and Taghreed Yahia Younis have noted that currently, 'honor-based' VAW has developed a broader horizon:

> A central aspect of violence and masculinity is violence against women, which ranges from physical, sexual and mental abuse to murder. The cultural option of taking women's lives has undergone some challenges and changes, yet, all in all…women and girls continue to be killed. Yet, ironically, while honour killings may have gone down in *some sectors*, the risk to women's lives has not diminished. In fact, it has magnified, since in addition to the cultural license to murder by blood relatives, husband too, who in the past would have been at risk of retaliation by the same blood relatives, have now joined the circle of

> potential killers. The traditional killing of women to preserve the honor of their kin group is now joined by killing in a so-called romantic setting. (Sa'ar and Yahia Younis, in Salhi, 2013, p. 17, emphasis in original)

Thus, the vicious circle widens. This brings us directly to our next section: rape, intimate partner violence, and family violence in the MENA region.

Other forms of VAW in Arab societies: Rape, Intimate Partner Violence and Family Violence

While scholars have noted a dearth of research on violence against women in the Middle East (Maziak & Asfar, 2003; Boy & Kulcycki, 2008), Human Rights Watch analyst Nadya Khalife has written a great deal about the reality on the street:

> [in the MENA region] Women are...reluctant to report domestic abuse, rape, or other forms of gender-based violence to authorities because of the difficulties they face in seeking redress...A few weeks ago, a young woman was allegedly raped in a restroom. The fact that she was treated like a criminal when she went to the police and that women in the Middle East are scared to report such crimes is the real moral outrage (*The Guardian*, January 29, 2010).

This sense on the ground is supported by a concrete '...lack of legal protections, public education campaigns, and services for victims' (Obeid, et al., 2010, p. 692). These researchers studied current attitudes toward wife beating among Lebanese university students (N=206). Specifically, they examined the associations between patriarchal attitudes, religion and childhood experiences of domestic violence with beliefs about wife battery. Several significant points emerged from their work. First, while there was a general inclination among the students to hold violent husbands responsible for their behavior, a strong degree of sympathy toward violent husbands was educed, and a 'remarkable' 40% of respondents agreed to, or were undecided about, the statement that the 'conditions of the husband's daily life play a major role in excusing his behavior' (p. 705). Following Haj-Yahia, (2000b), the authors noted that, 'These results are consistent with Arab sociocultural values that oppose wife beating in principle but nevertheless expect Arab women to support and understand the conditions of their husband (Obeid, et al. 2010, p. 705). Second, and as noted above, we see a reflection of more general attitudes in the region to so-called 'honor crimes' in that 26% of the students agreed or strongly agreed with the statement 'a sexually unfaithful wife deserves to be beaten' (p. 700).

Moving from students to the married population, in their study among low-income married women in Syria, Maziak and Asfar (2003) found current physical abuse in 23% of the sample. Tappis, Biermann, Glass, Tileva and Doocy. (2012) surveyed 486 married Iraqi women in Syria, and found that 30% reported a lifetime physical, verbal or emotional abuse. Douki et al. (2007) cited surveys that reported that at least one out of three women in several Arab states is beaten by her husband. Using data from the 1995 Egyptian Demographic and Health Survey, Diop-Sidibé, Campbell and Becker (2006) determined that 34% of women in the sample had been physically abused by her husband. Boy & Kulcycki (2008) found that of 59 studies located in a literature search on intimate partner violence in the Middle East, only 21 reported data on the prevalence of domestic violence or on perceptions of its justification, accounting for just 9 countries. They determined that intimate partner abuse is both pervasive and commonly accepted in the region. A further angle takes the pulse of the attitudes of the battered women themselves. Strikingly, Egyptian and Jordanian national data point to nearly 9 out of 10 ever-married women reporting as acceptable at least one reason for wife battering. And in a study looking at attitudes toward domestic violence in Jordan, Al-Nsour et al. (2009) found an 'alarmingly' high approval of wife beating among women in their sample. Thus, recalling data on 'honor-based' violence noted above, intimate partner violence in Arab/Islamic regions is not only widespread (as it is throughout the world); perhaps even more troublingly, it is quite well culturally ingrained, including among women.

Regarding women's attitudes toward physical abuse, Boy & Kulczycki (2008) found that culturally induced self-blame constitutes a major part of the picture of violence toward women in the Middle East. These researchers noted the data derived from five small-scale studies on women's beliefs about IPV. Among Israeli Arab women, agreement rates for justification of abuse in the case of a wife's marital infidelity reached 67-73% (Haj-Yahia, 1998, 2000); refusal to obey or nagging the husband, behaving in a way that causes a sense of family dishonor, poor care of the children and poor food preparation were other factors that Arab women throughout the Middle East considered reasonable precipitants for domestic violence (Boy & Kulczycki, 2008).

Family Violence

As noted above, in the Middle East, violence against Arab women perpetrated by extended family is prevalent. Thus, Morse, Paldi, Egbarya and Clark define "family violence' as gender-based violence against women perpetrated by any family member, including an intimate partner' (2012, p. 20). These researchers report that family violence constitutes a considerable health burden in the Middle East. Women in Jordan have an average 32-43% lifetime prevalence of IPV (Government of Jordan & ORC Macro, 2008, cited in Morse et al., 2012). Non-intimate partner family violence makes up 26% of VAW in this region, and has been linked to a highly significant increase in likelihood of IPV (Boy, 2008; Clark, Bloom, Hill & Silverman, 2009, cited in Morse et al., 2012).

Articulating the notion that the 'experiences, attitudes, and beliefs of abused [Arab] women' from the Middle East are poorly understood, Morse et al. (2012) investigated family violence among Jordanian women. These researchers did a thematic qualitative analysis of the perceptions of domestic violence on twelve focus groups among seventy married, divorced or widowed women. The five themes identified in the study show a range of ways in which gender-based family violence is implicated in health problems. Also revealed was the manner in which Jordanian female patients may keep the violence a secret.

The participant-perceived causes of gender-based family violence that emerged in Morse et al. (2012) were consonant with the themes that are discussed in this volume. For instance, male family members were expected to control – to the point of physical abuse - their female relatives who rejected culturally prescribed sexual norms:

> The father gave the son the right to control...he keeps telling his son: 'You are the man of the family when I am not at home, you should watch your sisters.'... The boy starts to dominate his sisters first, and when he gets married controls his wife and daughters (FG 5, P1, Morse et al., p. 22).

and:

> The brother...can do everything he wants, he is the man...he is the eldest one, even if he is only 10 years old. He could have the right to beat his 20-year-old sister if she went out with boys... (FG 10, P2, Morse et al., 2012, p. 22).

This male entitlement is not an isolated vestige of the past. Before us lies a current and culturally acceptable exemplar of conduct, strikingly reminiscent of Suad Joseph's ethnographic work with Lebanese Arabs, which took place more than four decades prior to this interview.

Salhi (2013) writes of the issue of defining violence against women. She notes cultural perceptions of VAW, and a widespread acceptance of verbal abuse and bullying that is found throughout the Arab world:

> In many Muslim countries in general and in the MENA region in particular, certain forms of violence are not seen as being violent acts such as verbal abuse and intimidation especially by intimate partners and/or by family members... It is a fact that verb abuse in such cases is considered a legitimate and mild method of correcting women and children (Salhi, 2013, Kindle edition).

Like Morse's work cited above, this account, too, is quite current, and reflects an ongoing reality in Arab societies. Notably, Salhi emphasizes that the VAW in the MENA region may be perpetrated by family members other than the intimate partner. We will now consider some specific circumstances under which family violence may occur in the Arab world.

Pregnancy, Infertility and VAW

In an investigation of reproductive health and IPV in Jordan, Jo Clark discussed the interlacing of violence against women and pregnancy:

> Second, forms of IPV were associated to some degree with family size and more substantially with pregnancy intention. This suggests that health providers need to be made aware of the potentially violent, controlling environment within which some women become pregnant, or attempt to avoid it (in Ennaji and Sadiqui, 2011, p. 186).

Infertility or the production of female children has been noted above to be considered a major failing when it occurs among Arab women. This, too, was demonstrated in the narratives of Morse et al. (2012), where such a 'failing' was associated with physical violence against women:

> When I married him and I started giving birth to my daughters, his family nagged him to remarry, and whenever they tell him that, he gets angry and starts beating me (FG 4, P2, p. 22).

In addition to describing intimate partner violence, the above narrative alludes to the complex dynamics of family-based violence ('whenever they tell him that, he gets angry and starts beating me'). The husband in the story is being pushed by his family of origin to enter into polygamy, a scenario of which we have taken note earlier, and his response is to abuse his wife. Here is another hint as to how the cultural acceptability of polygamy figures into the larger picture of violence against women.

In the above descriptions, extended family served as goads, or triggers, for violence against women. Morse et al. (2012) also found that this violence was frequently perpetrated by the extended family members themselves:

> I was humiliated from him...His sister used to beat me [because she covered my husband's and my expenses]...Once she hit me with a wooden stick while I was breast feeding my baby. And once my husband's sister and mother locked the door on me and started beating me both of them. He was sitting outside the room listening to me screaming. He didn't do anything (FG 6, P1, p. 24).

In this narrative, the male intimate partner is a bystander while the *female* extended family members are the violent actors. This is not an unusual scenario in traditional societies in general (see above section on India) and the Arab Middle East in particular (see al-Krenwi, 2014).

The 'honor crimes' discussed above also showed up in Morse et al.'s (2012) investigation. For instance:

> My husband's unmarried brother was sometimes coming and asking for a cup of tea. When my husband came and saw his brother sitting, he started slapping me and once he pulled me outside the house to his car where he wanted to get some gasoline for burning me...(FG 14, P3, p. 24).

The 'honor crime' in the text above prefigures the next one in this volume, the falsely accused wife in Al-Krenawi's work noted later in this chapter. Seeking assistance for such violence was reported in Morse et al. (2012) as a spur to greater violence:

> ...He bought a new set of knives, he tried them on his wife... he cut her skin, all over her body. (FG, 5, P4, p. 24).

The participants in Morse et al.'s (2012) study felt that their legal rights against family violence were extremely limited, and, moreover, that the enforcement of any such rights was negligible:

> There are...organizations [in Western countries] but here, there isn't any. Besides, how could the woman go to anyone? (FG 8, P2. p. 24).

and:

> The law is against you; what does the law do when the man slaps you and when you have filed a complaint against him? Maximum he will have to sign a paper that he will not repeat that, but the moment you go back home he will slap you again because he is not scared. What would the law do to him!... We will be blamed and it would not be accepted...for a woman [to] complain against her husband. (FG 14, P3, p. 24).

Three significant points arise from this report: One, the communal perception, at least from the point of view of the female participants, is that the blame for family violence in the Arab community will always fall on the female victim; two, the participants feel a strong sense of helplessness vis-à-vis family violence in their society; and three, that the participants believe there to be a lenient juridical stance toward family violence in the Arab states. Both of the first two issues parallel the expressions voiced by the participants in Al-Krenawi's work among Bedouin-Arab women in southern Israel (see chapter five), and the third has been touched upon in an earlier section in the current chapter.

Case Example

A case example with a number of relevant elements will serve to illustrate the degree to which the concept of 'honor' is embedded within Arab society, and in fact strongly colors notions of emotional health in that culture. In a paper on integrating cultural rituals into family treatment, Al-Krenawi (1999) describes a male Arab patient who was diagnosed with paranoid psychosis by an attending psychiatrist after the patient complained of somatic distress, inability to work, and persistent thoughts pertaining to his wife's (purported) sexual liaison with an extended family member. The wife denied such a relationship and reported that the husband had begun to hit her in his rage around the suspicion. The couple desired to consult with a traditional healer, a meeting encouraged by the treating therapist, and the healer suggested the intervention of a second healer who would conduct a traditional fire ritual known as *bisha*. Once initiated, this second healer informed the husband: *Ardaak Abiath*! ('Your honor is white!' that is, 'Your wife is not guilty of sexual impropriety!') (p. 67). The husband documented the session on tape to be produced as proof for his tribe, and the two returned home. Shortly thereafter, it was reported to the therapist that the husband went back to work and the domestic violence ceased.

This case example reveals a great deal about the dynamics of 'honor' in Arab society and, specifically, how the concept is tightly tied up with notions of sexuality and personal well-being. The following deconstruction of the case will clarify these points.

In the case at hand, an Arab husband and father of five presented with body weakness, loss of appetite, sleep disruption and intense preoccupation with the thought that his wife was sexually involved with a distant male relative. From the beginning, the extended family figured prominently in the picture: the patient's parents had seen a man near the patient's house in the late hours of the evening, and together with their son concluded that the wife was having an affair. Thus, the suspicion was introduced by family members, and the 'transgression' was framed as an assault upon familial, tribal and personal honor. Reporting that his 'honor' had been offended, the husband explained that this impelled him to beat his wife. He further articulated, 'I do not know where to put my face from the people', disclosing in metaphoric terms his powerful sense of shame vis-à-vis his tribe.

As the patient rejected the medications he had been prescribed for paranoid psychosis, there was no chance that either his shame or his suspicions could be effaced or even weakened by making use of them. Indeed, as we read above, only the culturally ordained ritual of *bisha* succeeded in removing the honor-based preoccupation of indignity from the mind of this patient. With documentation in hand, he was able to return to his social group, chief among them his parents, and present a 'clean bill of health' regarding both marital and familial honor, and his psychological state of being. In this way, the honor of the patient, of the patient's parents, and indeed of the patient's entire tribe was 'cleansed.' A consequent cessation of both symptoms and abusive was reported.

Our vignette tells us a great deal about the way in which personal (male) and familial honor are intertwined with mental health in the Arab region. But it also clues us in to the ways in which women's mental health is approached and managed in the Arab world.

Not only the husband, but also the wife in this case study is in clear distress. She is the victim of intimate partner violence, and has been accused of adultery, a crime with massive legal, social and emotional repercussions that she vehemently and consistently denied. (The progression of the story as set out by the both the husband and wife leads us to wonder if this instance of VAW was truly triggered by the suspicion, or that, as N. Singh has discussed, noted in chapter two, this is a mis-named honor-based crime that really masks ongoing VAW. In any case, while the wife is described as 'depressed', the author notes that 'more attention [in the sessions] was given to the husband's frustration. This was culturally demanded' (p. 67). While the therapist took pains to listen to both the husband and wife, he was culturally obligated to pay greater attention to the distress of the former

– despite the fact that the husband was actively beating his wife. Had he not done so, the author implies, he would not have been permitted to join the family system, and, far from failing – treatment would have never begun. This dynamic is a salient one in Arab treatment situations, reflective of broader views on the value and management of women's emotional distress. Below, we will explore more specifically the constructions of emotional distress in the Arab region.

Constructions of emotional distress in the Arab region: Male vs. Female

In line with previous investigations found in our chapter on Arab society, Seif El Dawla noted, 'It is one of the basic principles of Arabic and Islamic principles that the man has the major responsibilities in making important decisions' (in Okasha & Maj, 2001, p. 209). Here, we see a bedrock foundation for the workings of agency among Arab women: the express approval of a father or husband is required for a life direction to be taken. That the decision to seek professional help for emotional distress is made by the men in the Arab family may be considered, then, fairly expectable (Hamdan, 2009). As such, the gatekeepers to mental health treatment are the individuals with the most at stake in keeping intact the male-privileged, patriarchal structure of Arab society. While mental health intervention does not necessarily entail a destabilization of the existing familial structure (see chapter eight for more on this), clinical work that is not culturally competent in fact may portend just this outcome. Further, as 'anxiety and depression among Arab women may be considered part of their femininity' (Dwairy, p. 118), these disorders may be 'written off' as unworthy of treatment. Moreover, it has been noted that Arab women themselves seem to address their mental health needs last, only after those of their children and husband are adequately managed (Okasha et al., 1994, cited in Dwairy, 1998).

Significantly, education does not appear to have much of a mediating influence on this gender differentiation in mental health treatment. In point of fact, the converse seems true: the phenomenon can be traced back to Arab parents' mental health treatment choices for their children. Dwairy (1997b, cited in Dwairy, 1998) found that parents' educational levels were directly related to the number of male, but not female children engaged in psychotherapeutic work in his clinic in Palestinian areas in Israel. As the level of parental education rose, so did the number of boys in treatment:

no such correlation was found among the girls, who were referred by better-educated parents at a rate of one to five, compared to boys. It seems, then, that the gender-privileging noted by many researchers (Joseph, 1996; Abu-Lughod, 1986; Al-Krenawi, 2014) begun very early in life continues throughout the life course.

Khawla Abu-Baker (2005) has noted in her psychotherapeutic work with Arabs in the Middle East that Arab society provides two different ways of measuring and managing the emotional distress of male and female family members. Thus, when Arab women feel distress and seek support, they are considered 'unfortunate creatures in need of protection from their parents or their extended families' (p. 106). Contrariwise, an Arab man will typically receive assistance from his social group in bringing about an alleviation of his distress. This can take place in the most intimate of relations. For instance, if, for whatever reason, the wife of an Arab man refuses to cohabitate with him, she will be pressured by the community to modify her behavior. If this stratagem fails, the man will be encouraged to divorce her (a step with severe repercussions for the woman, including loss of her social status, money for basic living expenses, and oftentimes custody of her children. See Al-Krenawi & Graham, 2004). If the obverse situation obtains, however, and a man fails to have sexual relations with his wife (either willfully or by virtue of impotence), the community will typically censure the *wife*, and insist that she maintain a stance of 'mastoura' that is, stoicism, for the sake of the 'honor' of her husband and family (Abu-Baker, 2005). In fact, divorce in the case of male discontent is only one of the culturally acceptable options (for men) in Arab society: entering into polygamy is another. Scholars have written extensively on the growing phenomenon of polygyny in Islamic communities (Al-Krenawi, 2013). Earlier in this chapter, we noted a narrative in which the push for polygyny figured into intimate partner violence. Below, we examine this choice, and consider further ways in which it affects the mental health of Arab women.

Polygyny and Arab women's mental health

Al-Krenawi (2013) writes that while polygyny is found throughout the world, the practice is especially prevalent in heavily patriarchal regions such as the Middle East, where survival has traditionally hinged on ties to the community, the family and the tradition of the extended culture. Polygyny is common in Africa, Asia and parts of Europe; sub-Saharan Africa has the greatest prevalence, with a rate of higher than 10% in more than twenty-five states (Patil and Hadley, 2008). Islamic law stipulates that a man may be married to up to four wives at any given time, with the proviso that he supports them financially in an equitable manner (Khasawneh, Hijazi, Salman, 2011). Douki et al. (2007), considering the reception of polygyny by Muslim women in the Arab world, note that while Moslem women generally experience anxiety and fear around the threat of polygamy, the fact that it is religiously permitted dissuades them from its outright rejection (p. 184). Gregg Strauss (2012) tackles the issue of polygamy from the vantage point of ethics. Ultimately positing two possibilities for revamping the structure – and thereby the morality – of polygamy, the author sets out that:

> ...polygamy, as traditionally conceived, is morally objectionable because it precludes genuine equality between spouses. In traditional polygamy, only one person may marry multiple spouses. This central spouse divides him or herself among multiple spouses, but each peripheral spouse remains exclusively devoted to the central spouse. With this hub-and-spoke structure, even a perfectly virtuous central spouse has more rights and fewer obligations than each peripheral spouse. Moreover, a central spouse has more control over the family than each peripheral spouse. These inequalities are structural features of traditional polygamy, not merely contingent vices of modern polygyny (Strauss, 2012, p. 516).

Changing course from inequalities to legalities, there exists a heated and global debate on using legislation to attempt to control polygyny. In locales in which polygynous practice is recognized as a legitimate religious expression, states' efforts to regulate it run up against a veritable mountain of defense. It has been asserted by some religious leaders that the question should not even be considered under the domain of civil society (Al-Krenawi, 2013).

The persistence of patriarchy has been asserted to be at the heart of polygyny. Tertilt (2005) points to the pronounced inefficacy of anti-polygyny legislation, and suggests, in line with a number of scholars cited in this volume, that polygyny would die a natural death if the patriarchal stranglehold on female decision-making and financial security were to be loosened. Yamani (2008), too, reported that Arab women are culturally regulated in myriad ways that ensure their dependence upon men (cited in Al-Krenawi, 2013). Further support for this idea comes from El-Islam (in Al-Issa, 2000), who in discussing the status of Arab women 'emphasizes submission and dependency as important feminine attributes in the upbringing of girls' (p. 123). This dependence directly impacts on Arab women's sense of self. Below, we shall see how it is manifested in Arab women's responses to polygyny.

An accumulating body of research indicates that women experience more psychological distress in polygynous marriages compared to monogynous marriages (Khasawneh, Hijazi, and Salman 2011; Ozkan et al., 2006, Abbo et al., 2008; Al-Krenawi and Graham, 2006; Al-Krenawi, Graham, & Al-Krenawi, 1997; Al-Krenawi, Graham, & Slonim-Nevo, 2002, cited in Al-Krenawi, 2014; Al-Krenawi, 2013). Particularly germane to this volume, in which traditional healing treatments are reviewed (see chapter seven), in their study on psychological distress among users of traditional healing practices in eastern Uganda, Abbo et al. (2008) found that married women who had a co-wife reported more psychological distress than those without a co-wife. The authors discuss the possibility that polygamous relationships are more stressful to women than monogamous relationships.

Researchers who work among the Bedouin community in southern Israel write:

> Those who argue against polygyny are uncertain about how to respond to it. Some cite education and time as the solution. Others feel helpless and hope that change will come from without. A few express ambivalence, and state that they are powerless to produce change. While they recognize the harmful aspects of the practice and say they would choose differently, they cannot see how it is possible to contest the powerful forces of the society. In a community in which the woman's role is to be married and a mother, polygyny may be preferable to remaining single, despite the hardships that accompany it. Perhaps, they say, it is better to learn how to live with it. (Slonim-Nevo, Al-Krenawi, & Yuval-Shani, 2008, p. 205, cited in Al-Krenawi, 2014).

In this report of the female Arab experience of polygamy we read of the 'submission and dependence' to which researchers who study Arab women repeatedly refer. As outlined in chapter one, these twin topoi are rooted, according to Joseph (1996), in the patriarchy that persists in the Arab family. Growing from there, it manifests itself in resignation to painful, powerful realities, and a stance of helplessness in the face of overwhelming societal dictates. Thus, we see something akin to a state of learned helplessness (Seligman, 1975). Indeed, Chaleby (cited in El Dawla, in Okasha & Maj, 2001) links culturally driven passivity (i.e., males making all major life decisions) to the learned helplessness model of depression. This echoes Racy (1980), who described a pervasive passivity among his Saudi female patients:

> ...much effort is required to break through the barriers of somatization and passivity in order to get any specific picture of that particular patient's life, her concerns, and her tribulations' (p. 214).

Again we see the pairing of two of the major culturally driven emotional issues among women in the Arab world: somatization behavior and culturally fueled passivity/depression. A similar paradigm was offered by Abu-Baker (2005) in her depiction of the *'mastoura,'* the lauded stoic Arab woman who in dignity and silence accepts her 'fate.' This stance appears to have quite an unremitting quality: it has been reported among Lebanese Arab women in a recent volume on gender and diversity in the MENA region:

> [Lina] Khatib concludes that there is a need to focus on changing the systems and perceptions that trap women in a culture of passivity and self-denial (Salhi in Salhi, 2013, Kindle Edition)

Forced/Early Marriage in the Arab region

Arab women in the Middle East typically marry on the basis of familial, rather than personal considerations (Abu-Rabia Queder, 2007; Al-Krenawi & Graham, 2004; Al-Haj, 1987). Commensurate with the patriarchal nature of Arab society, marriages are arranged by male members of the extended families, and early marriages are not infrequent (Dwairy, 1998). These cultural traditions have survived modernity in the Arab region, and, both directly and as mediated through the marriage itself, impact on the mental – and physical - health of Arab women in the Middle East. On this topic, one scholar notes:

> Many women are forced to marry husbands they do not like or love...some of them find satisfaction after their marriages, while many others bury their romantic wishes and invest in the new roles as wives and mothers. Often, they identify with the oppressive norms and values from which they suffered and take part in an oppressive education of their children (Dwairy, 1998, pp. 181-182).

Dwairy is here spotlighting the female identification with patriarchal premises that have been discussed in earlier sections of this volume. As many scholars have alluded to in these pages, the work of patriarchy is not accomplished by men alone; women collude with the system and act as its representatives. Below, we will see this in the context of FGM/C.

We have clarified in the sections above on honor-based violence in the Arab world that arranged/forced marriages in this region can be a conduit to and justification for violence against women. While arranged marriages in and of themselves have not been proven to be categorically harmful to women, the imposition of this custom, with violent outcomes in the wake of its rejection, is highly detrimental to the emotional and physical wellbeing of women. Women in the Arab region, subject as they are to an environment of persistent patriarchy, are at particular risk for this form of abuse.

FGM in the Arab region

WHO estimates that 125 million women alive today have been cut in rituals of FGM. The great majority of these women live in Africa and the Middle East. Yotam Feldner (2000) refers to the possibility that this 'might be a phenomenon of epidemic proportions in the Arab Middle East' (p.7). Though found nowhere in the Koran, among the Muslim communities there is a common understanding that FGM/C is an Islamic practice recommended by the Prophet Mohammed.

FGM and Arab women's mental health

Al-Krenawi and Wiesel-Lev (1998) studied attitudes toward FGM/C among Bedouin Arabs of the Negev. With respect to the degree to which this ritual is embedded in Negev Bedouin culture, they noted that

> The circumcision ritual itself is inextricably associated with key Bedouin-Arab constructions of womanhood...Notions of spiritual purity are involved, which link directly to readiness for the attendant female-constructed responsibilities of being a mother and wife...while the ritual is imagined by outsiders to be nothing more than a relatively harmless ritual initiation... as practiced by the Bedouin-Arabs, [it] is often a euphemism for female mutilation (pp. 2-3).

Asali et al. (1995, cited in Al-Krenawi and Wiesel-Lev, 1998) reported that clitoridectomy is the most widespread form of FGM among this population; as such, the suppression of female sexuality is also at play.

Two distinct but highly related responses to FGM were expressed by these Bedouin women. Some subjects made body-image comments along the lines of, 'who owns my body, me or my husband?' and 'I felt something stolen from my body' (p. 7), while other participants made statements on the order of 'I would not be a good wife [without the ritual]' (p. 7). As being a 'good wife' constitutes the crux of self-identity for women in the Arab region, damage to that role is felt as both excruciating and highly anxiety-provoking; a husband may choose to take subsequent wives if he considers his wife lacking (see above). Complicating matters further, the practice of FGM itself may encourage polygyny, in that sexual problems are likely sequelae.

Finally, issues of female agency here loom large. On a certain level, at least, FGM falls within the 'women's realm.' That is, men are not involved in the actual ritual. Thus, anthropologist Van der Kwaak (1992, p. 785, cited in Al-Krenawi and Wiesel-Lev, 1998) has asked: 'What if the women concerned have a different perception...What if they do not want to be enlightened'? We will return to this question writ large in the conclusion of this volume, but here we will note that Al-Krenawi and Wiesel-Lev (1998) took this into account in their culturally sensitive, multi-step approach to this topic. They suggested, first and foremost, that the clinician assume an unbiased yet forthright stance, not sidestepping the subject, and, indeed, broaching it. They also offered culturally competent policy approaches, including ensuring that clients perform the ritual under adequate medical conditions, raising the age for having the ritual performed, and providing explanations and choices for girls.

Salaheldin Elgousi takes another approach. This author explicitly couples FGM/C with patriarchy. Salaheldin Elgousi's view on lack of female agency in the MENA region was presented in chapter one. Here, we broaden the discussion of FGM/C in Arab societies by noting the researcher's opinion on this topic, which is based on her work among Egyptian women:

> This [male control over women] is clearly demonstrated when the mother takes the decision to subject her daughters to the FGM/C operation. In her view, in doing so she is providing the essential protection to her child against committing indecent behavior that may put her female chastity and her family's honour at risk... (Elgousi, in Salhi, 2013, p.188).

In other words, Salaheldin Elgousi sees in women's participation in FGM/C the literal embodiment of patriarchy: the male desire to sexually control women is channeled through the female desire to safeguard herself and her daughters, even to the point of inscribing that patriarchy on their very bodies.

Some judicial movement on FGM/C is apparent in the MENA region. We conclude this section with notice paid to such development. A physician in Egypt was convicted very recently of manslaughter in a landmark genital mutilation case that involved the death of a 13 year-old girl. It was Egypt's first FGM/C trial; the doctor was sentenced to two years in jail for manslaughter and three months for performing FGM/C. As well, his clinic was closed for one year. (*Israel News,*January 26, 2015).

Culture or Religion: What does Islam have to do with it?

El-Islam stressed the intersectionality of religion and culture in the Arab region when he wrote that, 'What is traditional and what is Islamic have been closely identified with each other in everyday life and in Arab interpersonal relationships' (El-Islam, in Al-Issa, 2000, p. 123). This applies as well to the area of VAW. Morse et al. (2012) report a telling narrative on the topic:

> An Egyptian on the farm slapped his wife…I asked him: 'why did you hit her?' He said: 'our traditions and customs say: when the woman does not do what the husband is asking for, she should be slapped.' I asked him: 'religion has said this?' He said: 'no, religion says: treat them well, but we have our traditions.' Here the tradition has the upper hand over religion and has become the stronger rule in our life. (FG 15, P1, p. 24).

Morse et al. (2012) concluded that their data implicated patriarchal culture, rather than Islam, in violence against women.

The author and educator Irshad Manji addresses the problem of disentangling the origin of 'honor-based' violence against women. She maintains that while the violence is not condoned or instigated by classic Islamic texts, this type of crime is frequently perpetrated by Muslim individuals, who may conflate cultural Islam with religious Islam. Hence the confusion, beginning in the Muslim world and reflected by the world at large (Manji, 2011).

Moving to specifics, Ammar (2007) has investigated the range of Islamic interpretations of wife beating. Concentrating primarily on Arabic-language texts, she found an array of views on the acceptability of the act. The author begins with Verse 34 of the Koran, the *Al Nisa* (on women) chapter:

> ...As to those women on whose part ye fear disloyalty and ill conduct (*nushuz*), admonish them, refuse to share their beds, and beat [*idribuhunna*] them (Ammar, 2007, p. 520).

Ammar then categorized Islamic thought on the issue of wife battery into four major schools: (1) Unregulated permission to beat a wife if she does not obey her husband; (2) Conditional permission to beat a wife as a last resort; (3) Considering verse 34 to represent an exception to the overall thrust in Islamic sources (thus implying that 'wife beating in Islam is permissible but not desirable'); and (4) Defining the Arabic word *idribuhunna* as something other than striking. For example, the root of the word has been alternatively understood to mean *condemning* (Ammar, 2007, pp. 519-523). The author contends that the first view is not generally propagated by major religious figures, that the second position is non-historic, that the third position is held today by many Muslims and that the fourth point is both well established and well known. In Ammar's view, all of these interpretations enjoy a certain degree of contemporary currency.

Ammar's above-reviewed legal positioning of Koran 4:34 is also taken up by Ayesha S. Chaudhry in *Domestic Violence and the Islamic Tradition.* Chaudhry wraps up her investigation of pre- and post-colonial Sunni Muslim textual scholarship on marital violence in the following manner:

> This critical survey of historical and contemporary Muslim legal and exegetical scholarship on marital violence in the context of Q. 4:34 reveals that there has been a marked shift in the interpretation of the subject. This transformation is due in part to a new, idealized cosmology that has caused Muslim scholars to adjust their expectations of the divine text and a just God. The juggling of competing patriarchal and egalitarian cosmologies has triggered creative and exegetical legal trends...Furthermore, the sophisticated hermeneutical strategies have redemptive potential for the Islamic tradition... however, in order for Muslim scholarship to be able to move beyond the egalitarian-authoritative dilemma, egalitarian readings of Q. 4:34 must be able to lay claim to religious authority. This in turn depends on the ability of Muslim scholars to allow the Qur'an to be a performative text, so that

> Muslims can struggle with and determine its contemporary meanings (Chaudhry, 2013, p. 22).

The conclusion that the Koran must be allowed to be experienced as a performative text in order to fulfill its contemporary redemptive capacity is in line with the Islamic self-awareness sought by Ayman Sikseck, a young Israeli-Arab author:

> Islam does not condone murder, nor does it allow the restriction of civil liberties, and yet we have raised a generation of criminals who consider murder to be a legitimate form of opposition, and the robbery of human rights from women and non-Muslims an acceptable consequence of war. Terrorism was never a child of Islam, but we have fathered it nonetheless, allowing it to thrive within us, steal our identity, and operate on our behalf. So-called Muslims are the world's new mafia, and Islam itself is the recurring murder victim: in Syria, and Iraq, and Nigeria, and Europe, where its core values and principles are being altered and rewritten (Sikseck, 2014, no pagination)

While Sikseck is here lamenting global terrorism perpetrated by 'so-called Muslims,' his words speak directly to the heart of the matter regarding Muslim violence toward Muslim women. Linking the nurturing of terrorism with the spawning of oppression of women, the noted author contends further that:

> Our outrage over the bigotry and generalization that characterize the west's [sic] discussion of Islam has rendered us too rigid to reevaluate our failures. And we have undoubtedly failed. Though, not precisely the failure we are often accused of. But rather an internal failure, a generations-long pattern of idle resistance to extremism, and a feeble work ethic in mending our volatile Muslim societies. *Long standing traditions of oppressing Muslim women through legal and familial means*, and allowing Jihadist ideology to thrive in our own backyards, have reduced our apologies to the West to laughable rhetoric (Sikseck, 2014, no pagination, italics added).

Sikseck here renders a plea for Muslim self-critique on a community- and nation-wide level. He turns to 'enlightened Muslim leaders'; that is, those who are at this very moment choosing which of the four approaches set out by Ammar (2007) will be dominant, which of the cosmologies presented by Chaudhry will be engaged, and, indeed, precisely how Muslims will proceed into the post-modern future.

Conclusion

In this chapter, we have taken a close look at women's mental health in the Middle East, and arrived at a number of points. First, we have seen that the rates of prevalence among Arab/Islamic women for emotional problems that take up massive amounts of resources on a global scale (i.e., depression, anxiety and somatization behaviors) equal or surpass the rates that have been consistently found in large epidemiological studies among western women. Second, we have noted the urgent call for research on the mental health status among women in this region, reflecting the paucity of existing knowledge in this broad area. Third, we have attended to several cultural-specific factors (i.e., notions of female subordination, familial stigma and female/family honor codes) that affect the ways in which Middle Eastern society constructs its reality, and the ways in which women construct their reality vis-à-vis that framework. Finally, and crucially, we have explored a number of actions (VAW, HBV, HBM, FGM, polygamy) that strongly affect the mental and physical wellbeing of women in the Arab region. Here, too, we have noted the need for further research on how these acts affect women in the Middle East, and how best to pursue the amelioration of painful circumstances. These actions, endemic to much of the world, take on a unique hue in the context of the Arab world. In the next chapter, we take up another topic of global concern, but of particular manifestation in the Arab world: somatization and somatic symptom reporting.

Chapter 5
Somatization

'Every language grants us eloquence when it is time for help.' --Culture, Affect and Somatization, Laurence Kirmayer, 1984

Somatization has been conceptualized as the inclination to express physical distress in the face of psychosocial stress (Lipowski, 1988). A three-fold criteria set is frequently used to diagnose somatization: unexplained physical pain accompanied by psychosocial stress; patient attribution of physical illness, and the search for medical intervention (Clarke, 2008). Racy (1980) termed the behavior a kind of 'coded message' through which life difficulties are communicated in somatic language (Racy, p. 212). In this chapter, we explore the prevalence of somatization, as well as a range of opinions regarding both its diagnostic and empirical validity. Further, we engage with a related topic, that of *idioms of distress*, including somatic metaphors, whose presence has been documented in different cultures.

Prevalence

Large-sample size epidemiological studies have found prevalence estimates for somatization to hover around 20% (Gureje et al., 1997). Somatization has been found to be associated with depression and anxiety (Clarke, et al., 2008), and Barsky et al. (2001) report strong evidence of a gender disparity in its prevalence (Escobar et al. 1989; Escobar, et al., 1987; Escobar, et al., 1991; Kroenke, et al., 1997; cited in Barsky, 2001).

Primary care has been consistently found to be a core medical stage for somatization behavior. Clarke et al. (2008) found somatization behavior common in their large-sample size research with patients of Australian general practitioners, and Goldberg and Huxley (1992) found that a primary care physician was seen first by nearly two-thirds of individuals they studied who were eventually diagnosed as having a psychiatric illness. In a World Health Organization study that involved 14 countries and more than 25,000 patients, Gureje et al. (1997) found somatization to be a common problem in primary care settings across cultures, and that it was linked to significant psychological disability. In their massive epidemiological study, Kroenke (2003) found that one-quarter to one-half of primary and secondary care presentations fall into this category (Mayou, et al., 2005; Kroenke, 2003).

Somatization in the News: DSM Reconceptualization

Thus, it was the magnitude of the 'problem' of somatization that moved western researchers to pursue its reconceptualization. Not only mental health practitioners, but also medical doctors of all specializations are confronted by patients who complain of somatic pain that is difficult to make sense of from a medical point of view. Barsky et al. (2001) noted that while somaticizers are high utilizers of medical care, they and their clinicians are often left with a strong sense of dissatisfaction with care received (Kroenke, et al., 1997; Barsky et al., 2005; Lin, et al., 1991; Barsky et al., 1991). The enormity of the situation prompted careful consideration. And so we find that somatization is in the news. The notion that psychological distress may mask as physical symptoms, long-enshrined in western psychiatric lore and texts, has been recently and dramatically rethought – by none other than the bastion of the western psychiatric system itself. The diagnostic category of 'Somatization Disorders' was speculatively introduced in 1980 to the American Psychiatric Association's Diagnostic and Statistical Manual–III (APA, 1980). A host of problems related to its use has for many years spurred scholarly debate on its efficacy. These difficulties include ambiguous terminology, negative association with the term 'Medically Unexplained Symptoms' (MUS), DSM code confusion, difficult-to-use criteria sets, an overly wide criteria set for the diagnosis 'Undifferentiated Somatization Disorder' and a resulting tendency for clinicians to avoid the diagnosis altogether, for fear of incorrect ascription (Dimsdale, et al., 2013). Mindful of the pitfalls of the then-existing nomenclature, some of which encouraged an unhelpful mind/body dualism and all of which seem to float in a vague interstice somewhere between psychiatry and medicine, the DSM workgroup on Somatic Symptoms devised a new diagnostic category, Somatic Symptom Disorder (SSD). This new classification went into effect in 2013, in the newest version of the APA Diagnostic and Statistical Manual, DSM-V. A diagnosis of SSD is made when a patient reports persistent and clinically significant physical symptoms that occur in tandem with health-related thoughts, feelings and behaviors that interfere with his or her functioning. Hence, the diagnostic picture was widened to appreciate the degree to which these symptoms affect the overall life of the suffering individual (APA, 2013).

To Somatize or Not to Somatize: The Terminology Debate

Researchers, however, have noted that the very term 'somatization' reveals a western frame that is not shared by the global community. The concept has been traced to psychodynamic theories, in which repressed psychological conflicts manifest themselves in somatic symptoms, thereby taking the place of emotional expression. In this schema, the long-standing western mind-body split was upheld, and somatization problems were born (Kirmayer, 1984; Lipowski, 1988; Al-Issa, 1995). As early as 1997, Kirmayer and Weiss had recognized that the accepted classifications of somatoform disorders, which emphasized this division, were not in line with global findings. The bifurcation into 'psychiatric' and 'medical' disorders was quite artificial, it turns out, and served only as a kind of convenient category of miscellany (Weiss, Raguram, and Channabasavanna, 1995).

In fact, scholars have noted that the nosological issues on somatization do not end there. Kirmayer and Young (1998) enumerated several culturally related syndromes (Korean *hwa-byung*, Nigerian 'brain fag', South Asian *dhat*) that can result in culture-specific bodily complaints; these types of disorders, they noted, are completely missed by western symptom lists. Further, and perhaps more fundamentally, they suggest that culturally specific ailments should be understood as disorders unto themselves, and not as somaticized western emotional disorders (Mumford, 1996). Finally, as an alternative, they offer the idea that bodily complaints of frequent prevalence in fact might be related to particular western psychological ailments, but contribute in their own idiosyncratic ways to the illness trajectory. From this point of view:

> ...somatization cuts across the discrete categories of DSM...and the social and cultural processes that contribute to somatic modes of expressing distress can be understood...as modes of discourse or languages of suffering (Kirmayer and Young, 1998, p. 423).

Goldberg and Bridges (1988) outright rejected the notion that somatization was a disorder, and considered it a sort of joint mechanism in which both patient and clinician participate. Noting the extreme prevalence of the phenomenon, these researchers point out that physicians tend to encourage somatization by rewarding it with regard. Taking this point to its logical conclusion, Kirmayer and Young (1998) offer an arresting conceptual turnabout:

> ...somatization may be understood as a behavior of the clinician him/herself, who highlights, without taking into account the cultural connotations of such terms, only the somatic aspects of disorders (Kirmayer and Young, 1998, p. 423).

That the notion of somatization was the natural issue of a western, dichotomized view of the person is further elaborated by Dwairy (1998). He traces back the dualism to Descartes, and argues that the ancient and then later, non-western approaches were always more holistic, assuming a kind of mind-body unity. This unity extends to the symptom itself, as Barsky, et al. (2001) have noted: there is no physical symptom that is uni-dimensional; none that is not constituted of both body and mind elements.

Dwairy suggests three cultural points to consider with respect to somatization issues in the Arab regions: (1) non-western communities do not feature the kind of strong individuation of the self that is prominent in western regions, resulting in a body-centered identity; (2) fulfillment of basic, physical needs remain the preoccupation of many residents of non-western societies; and (3) authoritarian communities such as Arab ones hold individuals responsible for their thoughts and feelings, but assume that physical problems are outside the control of the person. Thus, treatment in these regions would be made readily available to sufferers of bodily ailments, while those in mental health distress might be expected to tolerate their pain (Dwairy, 1998). In a reversal of perspective that is reminiscent of Kirmayer and Young's above-mentioned views on 'clinician-encouraged' somatization, Dwairy (1998) contends that rather than much of the world engaging in 'somatization,' since the mid-seventeenth century and the advent of Cartesian logic, the western world has been inclined to 'psychologize' pain, to the detriment of the whole person. Kirmayer wrote of this detriment when he noted, following Sontag (1978), that "psychologization' has gone so far among some North American subcultures that it may lead to a tendency to blame victims for willfully causing their own somatic diseases' (Kirmayer, 1994, p.175).

Somatization Behavior across Cultures

Somatization behavior has been found to be quite ubiquitous across cultures (Kirmayer, 1984; Kirmayer and Young, 1998; Al-Issa, 1995). Indeed:

Somatization has been found wherever it has been sought and, worldwide, somatic symptoms are more common than emotional complaints as a way of presenting psychosocial distress' (Kirmayer, 1984, p. 161)

Nonetheless, the notion that somatization is more common among certain ethnic groups such as the Chinese (Kleinman, 1982), Hispanics (1990) and Japanese (Radford et al., 1989) was once predominant (Al-Issa, 1995). A theorized incapacity of some persons to verbally communicate psychological pain was put forward by some scholars. This purported inability was partially based on the finding that certain languages lack an equivalent word for particular psychological distress (e.g., depression in Chinese) (Al-Issa, 2001; Leff, 1973). While emotional expression is no doubt related to language, the heuristic value of this notion is seriously reduced by the fact that somatization is frequently reported in the Arab world, where the emotional lexicon is far from lacking (Al-Issa, 1995). Indeed, this language deficiency attribution has been roundly rejected by transcultural experts (Al-Issa, 2000).

Another version of this theory, however, has been promoted by a number of well-respected Muslim mental health practitioners (El-Islam, 1982; Okasha, Bishry, Khalil, Darwish, Seif Al-Dawla, and Shohdy, 1994). These scholars, based on work done by Shouby (1951), assert that in order to be taken seriously, Arabic speakers make use of the rhetorical tool of hyperbole – a tool that they posit is intrinsic to the language. Thus, the reasoning runs, Arabic-speaking patients are predisposed towards emotional expression and somatization. Al-Issa (2000) disallows this entire construct as purely conjectural.

It is now known that it is only the particular manifestations of bodily distress associated with emotional distress that vary across cultures (Hall, 2005). Beiser (2003) set this progression out clearly when he noted that initially, cross-cultural psychiatry spotlighted exotic 'culture-bound syndromes' (Yap, 1951), then moved to more nuanced depictions of cultural impact on symptoms, especially those related to affective disorders (see below). Beiser goes on to repudiate the 'Asians somatize, North Americans psychologize' maxim on the basis of research that revealed that First Nations, Southeast Asian and West African individuals do in fact use psychological terms – though with culture-specific nuances - to report depressive complaints (Beiser, et al., 1994).

From quite a functional point of view, somatic symptoms have been thought to play a role in social structuring. That is, they may serve as tools to spotlight social problems, connecting the person and his or her social and political spaces (Al-Issa, 1995). For instance, in his research in Arab

Gulf communities El-Islam (1982a, 1984) found that the failure (actual or imagined) of Qatari women in marital and maternal spheres was highly associated with somatic presentation. These ailments garnered a great deal of sympathy from family and medical workers, essentially reversing the expected outcome: no longer social failures, these women were 're-categorized' as somatic sufferers. In this way, the physical complaints of the women transformed their social identities. As persons living in a *sociocentric* (Adeponle et al., 2012) society, the social identities of Arab women throughout the Arab region take pride of place in their lived experience. This, as we shall see, yields a significant intersectionality of social identity and mental health for the Arab women in the Middle East.

Somatization and Affective Disorders

A large body of literature exists on the presentation of somatic symptoms alongside depression and anxiety. For instance, Amin, Hamdi and Abou-Saleh (in Okasha and Maj, 2001), found that among Arab patients, bodily complaints may substitute completely for depressed symptoms, that hard-to-describe psychological experiences were verbally expressed as unusual somatic sensations, and that somatic pains tended to be the initial and overwhelming complaint. Rather than complaining of anhedonia and sadness, Arab depressed patients have been found to report physical symptoms (El-Islam, et al., 1988). This presentation may be related to a number of factors, including medical attention paid to bodily complaints and stigma (Okasha and Maj, 2001). El-Rufaie, Al-Sabosy and Bener (1999) found a very high rate of somatic presentation among Saudi Arabian psychiatric patients, and Chaleby (1999) noted that a full 56% of 270 sampled Saudi Arabian patients somaticized emotional distress. Headache and feelings of dizziness were the top-ranking somatic complaints in this cohort. Saudi females were investigated by Racy (1980) as well, who found a great deal of somatization, which he maintained constituted a response to authoritarian contexts. In Racy's view, the Saudi women he studied unconsciously used bodily complaints to circumvent pervasive masculine control over their lives.

Bener et al. (2012) studied the comorbidity between somatization and stress and anxiety and depression in a primary-care population in Qatar. They found a similar rate of somatization of and depression, with stress higher among inpatients than outpatients. Stress disorders, depression, somatization and anxiety co-occurred at a higher rate in the study sample.

Somatization behavior tends to take place in particular contexts. Primary care has been called the 'central arena for the delivery of mental health services' (Kirmayer et al., 1993, p. 734). Noting the strong prevalence of somatization in primary care, these researchers investigated the impact of several somatization behaviors on the rate of physician recognition of anxiety and depression in family practice. They found that somatic presentations, in contrast to hypochondriacal fears and medically unexplained somatic symptoms, decreased physician recognition of these affective disorders.

The management of symptom reporting and somatization is further complicated by the culturally created frame in which patients approach clinicians:

> People bring symptoms and predicaments to their doctors, not just diseases or disorders. These predicaments may contribute to the cause, course, and outcome of a specific disorders. Because these predicaments are socially constituted, they will differ across social and cultural contexts, giving rise to potentially important differences in the nature of psychopathology (Gone and Kirmayer, 2010, p.90).

In point of fact, then, somatization behavior is colored in important ways by the specific circumstances in which it occurs. Below, we consider the intersectionality of somatization and affective disorders in a particular space: among women in low- and middle-income countries.

Somatization, Women and Affective Disorders in Low- and Middle-Income Countries (LMIC)

Across cultures, females are more likely than males to describe coterminous somatoform disorders and anxiety or depression (Kessler et al., 2003; Mirza and Jenkins, 2004, cited in Shidhaye, Mendenhall, Sumathipala, Sumathipala and Patel, 2013). In consideration of this fact, Shidhaye et al. (2013) investigated the co-morbidity of somatoform disorders with anxiety and depression among female patients in low- and middle-income countries (LMIC). They included 21 studies in their review of two databases, and concentrated on community and primary health care-based research. These authors found that women who present with somatic complaints typically do not relate these to emotional distress. Instead, they construe their distress in terms of day-to-day challenges, and also provide an array of interpretations of the pain (Patel, et al., 2008a, cited in Shidhaye et al., 2013). Interestingly, while 'tension' is not offered as an explanation for somatic symptoms, in their stories women made ample reference to psychosocial distress (Patel et al. 2008b, cited in Shidhaye et al., 2013, p. 5). The researchers concluded that in community and primary health care settings, an association exists for women between somatization disorders, depression and anxiety:

> Most studies showed an association of SD [somatization disorder] and depression and anxiety alone or together; some studies demonstrated this relationship with somatic symptoms...About one-fourth to one-third of women who present with SD/somatic symptoms were diagnosed with depression and/or anxiety...Our findings are consistent with the results of studies from high-income countries (Wessely et al., 1999), suggesting that the association of SD with depression and anxiety among women is cross-cultural (Shidhaye et al., 2013, p. 6).

Conclusion

In this chapter we tackled somatization from a number of angles, even questioning its very construction. As considerations of culture constituted the warp and woof of this inquiry, it is fitting that we conclude with some words from Laurence Kirmayer upon the Jubilee year of the *Journal of Transcultural Psychiatry*. In his role as chief editor of the journal, Kirmayer discussed its conceptual trajectory, beginning with viewing cultures as '... self-contained local worlds...' and moving towards approaching culture as:

> '...based on social processes of identity construction' that result in 'creative transgression, contestation, and transformation...psychiatry is now part of transnational flows of information that are used by professionals, institutions, and individuals to refashion identities in health and illness (Kirmayer, 2013, pp. 4-5).

Such a perspective moves us toward the mending of age-old cleavages, whether represented by images of East-West or mind-body.

Costa and McCrae (1985) offered a multi-dimensional model of somatic pain, and suggested that mental health practitioners 'move beyond naïve realism and psychiatric dichotomies' (p. 26) in understanding bodily distress. Barsky et al. (2001) remind us that '*all* symptoms are 'real,'' (p. 272, italics in original) and enjoins the clinician to make a vigorous attempt to grasp the unique meaning of each patient's symptoms. Along these lines, rather than dichotomizing symptoms, and thus the person, Engel (1977) suggests that the interpenetration of the emotional, physical and cultural aspects of help-seeking behavior become the subject of investigation. Such a research direction would be inclined to respect the poignant fact that 'human suffering is cut from one cloth' (Kirmayer, 1984, p. 175).

In the same vein, Beiser (2003) offers a plea for 'investigations aimed at getting behind the veil of culture to glimpse the shared anxieties, aspirations, and hopes that transcend the gloss applied by culture' (Beiser, p.158). Interestingly, this plea, complete with its veil metaphor, echoes that made by the anthropological and literary scholars noted in the conclusion to this volume. In those cases, of course, the hope is that Arab/Muslim women specifically will be viewed in their actual fullness of lived experience. In both cases, though, the scholars look toward a future in which a '...constant recognition of our common humanity, a humanity subjected to different forces and expressed in different registers' (Abu-Lughod, 2013, p. 227) is realized. It is with this thought that we now turn to the transcultural language of idioms of distress: metaphors and proverbs.

> 'In some linguistic communities, nothing rings so true as the simplicity of an appropriately used proverb' -- Bryan B. Whaley (1993)

> 'Dichos son el juicio de su gente' ('Dichos –Proverbs-are the wisdom of your people') -- Hispanic/Latino Proverb, from Aaron Aviera (1996)

> 'If you really want to understand Ayuveda [traditional Indian healing]... the place to begin is your stomach.' — in Nichter, *Coming to Our Senses: Appreciating the Sensorial in Medical Anthropology (2008)*

Chapter 6
Idioms of Distress, Proverbs and Metaphors

Three decades ago, medical anthropologist Mark Nichter coined the term *idioms of distress* to describe the ways in which a sense of affliction is communicated in different cultures:

In any given culture, a variety of ways exist to express distress. Expressive modes are culturally constituted in the sense that they initiate particular types of interaction and are associated with culturally pervasive values, norms, generative themes, and health concerns (Nichter, 1981, p. 379).

These idioms vary across sociocultural groups, and are derived from the main metaphors and traditions of a given collective. For instance, symptoms may be clustered into syndromes in different ways across groups, resulting in a diagnostic scheme that varies from culture to culture. As well, some cultures may be relatively inclined to use psychological terminology in their self-evaluations of wellbeing, whereas others may tend towards somatic representations of their bio-psycho-social state (Good, 1977, cited in Hinton & Lewis-Fernández, 2010).

Pointing to the heuristic value of the term, the Diagnostic and Statistical Manual of Mental Disorders (DSM-5) has added *cultural concept of distress* to its diagnostic framework: 'Cultural Concepts of Distress refers to ways that cultural groups experience, understand, and communicate suffering, behavioral problems, or troubling thoughts and emotions' (AMA, 2013, cited in Kohrt, Rasmussen, Kaiser, Haroz, Maharjan, Mutamba, de Jong, and Hinton, 2014, p. 366).

Nichter (2008) has situated the notion of a 'somatic idiom of distress' within the work of sensorial anthropology. Thus, he writes:

> Somatic idioms of distress refer to the ways in which visceral responses to distress communicate angst to significant others. Somatic sensations resonate within one's social universe whether consciously acknowledged or not. Somatic distress can also constitute an expression of collective ills (Frankenberg, 1986) when experienced as a form of somatic response to forms of oppression. In some cases, this visceral expression can serve as a form of protest, a 'weapon of the weak' (Scott, 1985), albeit a protest easily medicalized (Frankenberg, 1986; Scheper-Hughes, 1991). Attentiveness to visceral expressions of distress can also serve as an idiom of concern at the site of the body (Nichter, 2008, p. 166).

In his early work, Nichter (1981) wrote of the somatization that he found to be a central idiom through which distress was conveyed among Havik Brahmin women in the Indian community of South Kanara. These woman shared a number of life-course features with Bedouin Arab women, whose powerful use of metaphors and proverbs we will discuss below. Nichter noticed that in consultation with indigenous practitioners:

> The reporting of somatic symptoms was observed to take precedence over more descriptive statements indicative of affect states. Such states were rarely elaborated or dwelled upon, and discussion about affect was almost always initiated or followed up by concern shown about a somatic complaint (Nichter, 1981, p. 387).

Idioms of distress: Western as well as Eastern

Since Nichter's early work, multiple exotic idioms of distress have been reported. Hence, in their paper on idioms of distress among trauma survivors, Hinton & Lewis-Fernández (2010) take pains to note that idioms of somatic distress are not unique to non-western communities. The authors cite Strine and Hootman's (2007) work on the 'epidemic of 'lower back pain,' which is endorsed by as many as 26% of U.S. adults' (p. 2): Hinton & Lewis-Fernández continue that, 'This U.S. idiom of distress is characterized by a web of cultural associations, which include overwork (as in the trope, 'back-breaking labor'), general 'stress', and even moral failure (e.g., 'more than I can bear,' 'a monkey on his back,' 'spineless')' (p. 2). Further, 'These associations link work-related and interpersonal tension specifically to the back muscles via a process of somatization...' (p. 2; Hinton and Good, 2009, Kleinman et al., 1992, cited in Hinton & Lewis-Fernández, 2010). This somatic idiom of distress, which would be instantly recognizable to any American adult, has the potential, however, to turn into illness:

> Biological mechanisms are recruited for their expression and may result in chronic disease over time, especially in genetically or temperamentally vulnerable individuals. Back pain that results in inactivity, bad posture and excessive bed rest may yet develop into chronic muscle pathology (Hinton & Lewis-Fernández, 2010, p. 2).

Thus,

> ...behaviors and interpretations that originate as meaning-related expressions become *embodied*, and what starts out as an idiom of distress may end up also

being a 'disease,' a biologically encoded pathway with its own self-perpetuating pattern (Kleinman et al. 1978, cited in (Hinton & Lewis-Fernández, 2010, p. 2, italics added)

Just as an idiom of distress may transform into illness, it may not. In their investigation of somatic symptoms among female Japanese and Korean students, Saint Arnault & Kim (2008) underscored the distinction between idioms of distress and mental illness, and caution against a confusion of the terms. In a point that again harkens back to the Introduction, they write that while these idioms may indeed signal somatic or emotional disorder, they may just as likely 'be culturally coded ways of expressing social discontent' (p. 28). In fact, thirty years after his initial formulation, Nichter (2010) noted in a review that his original stance had been to argue:

> ...for an assessment of the range of possible ways in which different members of a population might express or enact various types, levels and intensities of distress, and the circumstantial factors favoring/disfavoring one culturally salient means of expression over another (p. 403).

In the same context, Nichter also wrote about the ways in which the concept of idioms of distress had taken hold in the world; following Abu-Lughod, we might call this the 'social life' of idioms of distress.

Lillian R. Furst's *Idioms of Distress: Psychosomatic Disorders in Medical and Imaginative Literature* (SUNY Press, 2003), for instance, represents one trajectory in the life-course of idioms of distress. There, she notes the definition of idiom offered by the Oxford English Dictionary: 'a form of expression, a construction, often having a meaning other than its grammatical or logical one' (Furst, 2003, p. 12). Furst hones in on the relationship between idiom and metaphor when she writes that:

> ...in its character as a construct, it denotes something newly created to fit a particular purpose... in its departure from...grammatical meaning...an idiom moves toward metaphor, a mode of speech that entails a figurative transference from one medium to another'(Furst, p. 12).

Idiom of Distress as Metaphor: Definition and Critique

Metaphor is at the heart of the definition of idiom of distress offered by de Jong and Reis (2010):

> an embodied symbolic language for psychosocial suffering that derives its legitimacy from its shared metaphors, meaning and understanding in a social group...its multilevel and multi-interpretable nature and its use of condensed symbols allow the individual to express and communicate suffering caused by different types of stressors that cannot otherwise be expressed in the local social-cultural-political context, due to the threat such expression would constitute to culturally dominant values and structures (p.302).

The notion of a relationship between idiom and metaphor has crystallized into a major critique of the concept of idioms of distress. Lee et al. (2007) turned our attention to 'the way in which labeling embodied emotional expressions as metaphors or idioms leads us to think of them as figurative, and not genuine...' (Nichter, 2010, p. 408), In response, Nichter points to his call for a sensorially engaged anthropology (Nichter, 2008a, 2008b). In this, he notes that 'the study of somatic idioms of distress demands more than a clever mind...It requires of the researcher...to engage in a somatic mode of attention that is reciprocal and humbling' (Nichter, 2010, p. 409). As metaphor plays a constitutive role in the framing of mental health among women in the Arab region, we now turn to a fuller account of both it and its counterpart, the proverb.

Metaphors

The word *metaphor* is derived from the Greek word meaning 'to transfer.' (Online Etymology Dictionary). Metaphors have been for centuries used in a wide range of stories intended to promote change (Cambell, 1988, cited in Guiffrida, 2007). In Langer's (1948) view, metaphor succeeds as a growth agent precisely because through it, novel information is 'transferred' to familiar frames of reference, thus reducing the difficulty in knowledge acquisition. Like proverbs, metaphors may be more than they seem: Abrahams (1968) held that the heart of metaphoric work lies in 'artfully disguising recommendations' (cited in Aviera, 1996, p. 77)

Due to its capacity to elicit growth, metaphors have been part of the therapeutic toolkit of western clinicians for at least a century (Barker, 1985, cited in Guiffrida, 2007). Such leading figures as Sigmund Freud, Rollo May, Carl Jung, Milton Erikson and Carl Rogers encouraged the use of metaphor in psychotherapeutic treatment (Guiffrida, 2007). Metaphor use in traditional healing goes back much further in time (Witztum, 1988).

Aviera (1996) wrote that Barker, in his *Using Metaphors in Psychotherapy*

(1985) offers a number of ways in which metaphors, including proverbs, may be used in clinical work. Describing the efficacy of metaphors as related to the fact that they 'are interesting, captivating, and flexible,' as an 'indirect' and 'veiled' form of expression, metaphors are experienced by the patient as non-confrontational (Aviera, p. 77). Barker goes on to argue that proverbs 'can be used to illustrate a point, suggest a solution to a problem, reframe problems...decrease resistance, plant ideas, increase motivation, and even build self-esteem...' (Aviera, 1996, p. 77).

Proverbs

Whaley (1993) has noted the large body of literature that points to the notion that 'a strategic use of language facilitates change' (p. 127) (Fisch, Weakland, & Segal, 1992; Grauf-Grounds, 1982; Haley, 1973, 1976; Norton, 1981, all cited in Whaley, 1993). The rhetorical features of metaphor have been singled out as notably therapeutic (Haley, 1976; Sullivan, 1985, 1986; Watzlawick, 1978, cited in Whaley, 1993). The study of the therapeutic benefit of proverbs, however, is still in its infancy.

The definition of the term proverb has been debated for centuries. Whiting (1932) wrote that 'there is nothing so elusive, so evasive, as the exact sentence, or group of sentences, which should constitute such a definition of proverb (Whiting, 1932, p. 273, cited in Whaley, 1993). Norrick (1985) offered that the proverb 'is a traditional, conversational, didactic genre with general meaning, a potential free conversational turn, preferably with figurative meaning (Norrick, 1985, p. 78, cited in Whaley, 1993).

Proverbs may be deceptive in their semantic simplicity. Nguyen, Foulks & Carlin (1991) note that western societies disparage proverbs, considering them too succinct and highly diffused among cultures to represent true wisdom. In sharp contrast to that view, these researchers maintain that the manipulation of proverbs demands high-level cognitive skills. They note that Haneck and Kibler (1984) asserted that the use of proverbs entails no fewer than four cognitive steps: recognition of the inapplicability of the literal sense of the proverb to the issue at hand; understanding that the proverb must in some manner apply to that very issue; the search for a 'figurative' meaning applicable to other similar situations; and finally, arriving at a sort of conceptual generalizability. This last is what allows for therapeutic growth (Nguyen, et al., 1991).

What is the actual mechanism by which proverbs fuel therapeutic movement? Nguyen et al. (1991) suggested that the key to proverbs' power is that they 'cloak anxiety-laden, raw conflicts in more abstract, and therefore more acceptable, symbolic form (Nguyen et al., 1991, p. 312). In his work on the rhetorical characteristics of proverbs, Whaley enumerates nine features that have been put forth as change-enhancing:

> (1) Proverb as analogy; (2) proverb as ambiguity; (3) proverb as contradiction; (4) proverb as enthymeme; (5) proverb as speech act; (6) sociability of proverbs; (7) the framing function of proverbs; (8) the poetic features of proverbs; and (9) the proverb as equipment for living. (Whaley, 1993, pp. 139-135)

Below, we will explore the use of proverbs among persons in the Arab region, as well as several other ethnic groups. In the process, we will note many traces of these basic characteristics.

Use of Proverbs by Ethnic Hispanic/Latino Peoples

Dichos are Spanish-language proverbs. Hispanic/Latino individuals throughout the world make use of *dichos* (Aviera, 1996). Zuniga (1991, 1992, cited in Aviera, 1996) used dichos in her treatment of Hispanic/ Latino college students to foster a sense of hope, and later, to manage resistance. Importantly, this was done with the conscious intention to draw 'upon a cultural perspective that can make this often foreign clinical situation less threatening' (Zuniga, 1992, p. 57, cited in Aviera, 1996, p. 76). Like the use of proverbs by ethnic groups noted below (Vietnamese and ethnic Arab), the culture-specific aspect of proverbs lends a great deal to the therapeutic environment, enabling the patient to tap into sources of wisdom in times of stress that are already part and parcel of their worldview.

Zuniga (1992, cited in Aviera, 1996) provided an example of a *dicho* that served such a purpose. In her case example, a female Hispanic /Latino student was the victim of IPV in a relationship that both her family and community expected to result in marriage. Echoing the case examples below in the section on ethnic Arab women, this student struggled with a 'cultural script' of pressure to become both wife and mother (p. 58). In the course of the treatment, the *dicho, 'Mejor sola que mal acompanda'* ('It is better to be alone than in bad company') (p. 58) was explored, serving as cultural affirmation that a healthy relationship was indeed valorized by her culture. Here, we see an instance of a proverb serving what Whaley (1993) and Barker (1985) considered a 'framing' function. That is, the proverb enabled the patient to re-frame her view of the expectations of her cultural heritage.

Aviera (1996) used *dichos* in his group work with Hispanic/Latino psychiatric patients. His interest in *dichos* was piqued when he noted the effect the presentation of the proverb had on the patient who offered it: this chronically mentally ill person became animated and focused. In essence, as much as the patient 'spoke' the *dicho*, it spoke for him – and of him. Aviera found that a group dedicated specifically to a discussion of the patient's cultural proverbs served many therapeutic goals. First, it granted legitimacy to their cultural heritage, and indirectly, to themselves within it. Second, it helped to draw to the fore feelings of low self worth (see section on ethnic Arabs below), hence creating a space for working on this issue. For instance, the *dicho*, '*Del arbol caido, todos hacen lena*' (From a fallen tree, everyone makes firewood') (Gkavab & Teschner, 1985, cited in Aviera, 1996, p. 80) were triggers for patients to discuss feelings of being misused, and abused. Here, the use of proverb as analogy is evident.

Generally speaking, and as noted by the author, insight-oriented therapy was beyond the purview of the population with whom Aviera worked (although the *dichos* technique did serve as a springboard for some insight-oriented discussion). Further, also discussed in the paper, these patients were unfamiliar with psychological language, having spent their lives on remote farms. Hence, these were not patients inclined to 'psychologize' their emotional distress. The findings, then, might be useful in planning treatment for different groups that are not highly immersed in the langue of western psychology.

Proverbs in the form of *dichos* have been presented here as a clinician-introduced therapeutic tool. In the next two sections, we will see examples of the clinical harnessing of the spontaneous expression of proverbs among Vietnamese and ethnic Arab patient groups.

Use of Proverbs by Ethnic Vietnamese Peoples

Traditionally, educated Vietnamese were expected to memorize volumes of classical Vietnamese proverbs (Dang Liem, 1969, cited in Nguyen, Foulks & Carlin (1991). Thus imbedded within Vietnamese culture are particular proverbs, and thus are they valued as a fundament of Vietnamese heritage. Nguyen et al. (1991) explored proverbs as psychological interpretations among ethnic Vietnamese. They found that the sampled individuals used proverbs in a way that demonstrated a psychological mindedness that was not obvious in other communication patterns in this ethnic group. The commonly acknowledged use of proverbs in Asia communities is noted by these authors, who emphasize that nonetheless, the *function* of the proverbs among this group is a topic that has been given short scholarly shrift. They maintain that among Vietnamese (and, perhaps, other Asian groups) proverbs are an important component of communication in that they serve as a conduit for empathy, as well as gently cut through thickets of dysfunctional defenses. In this context, we are considering the day-to-day use of proverbs between family members and close friends.

Like Al-Krenawi in his work with Bedouin-Arab patients, Nguyen et al. (1991) proposed that the generally somatic presentations of Vietnamese patients reflect their treatment setting: a biomedical clinic. That is, those who seek help in a medical venue expect to phrase their complaints in bodily terms. This, they contended, in no way indicates a lack of 'psychological mindedness' on the part of the sampled patients.

Nguyen et al. (1991) offered a number of examples of 'how a particular psychologically defensive posture was addressed in the proverbial rendition' (p. 314). For instance, they cite *'Ai o' trong chan, moi biet chan co ran'* ('Whoever sleeps in a blanket knows it has lice') (p. 314). The authors offer as an explanation for the proverb the hypothetical situation of a woman living with marital discord; a confidant might bring up this proverb in an effort to help her friend to 'air out the vermin-filled blanket' (p. 314). The thrust of the proverb use is psychodynamic: keeping pain under wraps is not good mental health practice. In this example, we may detect the mechanisms of proverb as speech act and sociability.

A second example offered by these authors illustrates an interesting point pertaining to somatic distress. One the face of it, the proverb *'Ai trong thay ma, moi biet dan ba an o't'* ('He who can see ghosts is able to know a woman is eating chili peppers') (Nguyen et al., 1991, p.314) conjoins highly disparate elements. The listener wonders where the proverb is going. Nguyen et al. (1991) inform us that in traditional Vietnamese culture, ghosts are considered actual, potentially visual, entities. Chili peppers are known to cause gastric upset, something that is also caused by a range of feelings that one might wish to hide. Further, common lore has it that women enjoy eating these peppers and that they become progressively more jealous as they eat them. Thus, the proverb yields the idea that 'someone [like me] who is psychic enough to see ghosts, is certainly perceptive enough to see that a woman [you] has indigestion [from guilt or stress]' (Nguyen, 1991, pp. 314-15). Hence, once again an everyday Vietnamese proverb transmits the message that the outcome of suppressing affect is bodily pain, and that the best course of action is to unburden oneself to an appropriate individual. This exemplar highlights the power of the poetic feature of the proverb, 'cloaking a recommended course of action in the garb of artful expression' (Abrahams, 1968a, cited in Whaley, 1993).

Use of Metaphors and Proverbs by Ethnic Arab Peoples

Amin et al. (2001) found that Arab patients used a variety of metaphors to describe depression. Not at all simple constructions, these were multidimensional phrases intended to describe changes in emotional states. For instance, the heart was considered the seat of actions: 'the fear is inside the heart'; 'the heart does not want to eat'; 'the heart is poisoning me.' Echoing medical anthropological work on somatic idioms of distress, these researchers put forth that an attentive examiner can tease out the relationship between these bodily metaphors and emotional distress. Further, they note that in his classic paper on transcultural aspects of dysphoria, Bebbington (1993)

> acknowledges that even English terms used to describe mental phenomena are based on somatic metaphors which disappear gradually, leaving the term hanging like the tip of an iceberg.' (Okasha and Maj, p. 106)

Thus, the universality of somatic metaphors has been colorfully and carefully limned.

Some researchers maintain that clients from the Middle East are inclined toward metaphoric language in their clinical presentations (Dwairy, 1998). Depression may be alluded to as 'dark life'; loneliness as 'I am the guardian of the wall'; anxiety in 'my heart fell'; and a sense of fearful, angry astonishment as 'my mind flew up' (Dwairy, p.168). It has been put forth that some languages are particularly metaphoric (Barakat, 1993; Hourani, 1991, cited in Dwairy, 1998). Metaphors, then, are made constant use of in cultures with these metaphor-laden languages; they become the key to communication.

In this regard, proverbs were noted to be highly salient in contemporary Arab medical institutional communications. A recent paper on the effects of the social status of the aged in Libya on their communication with young physicians (Wei, Mayouf, 2009) reported that elderly patients mainly used religious expressions and proverbs to describe their ailments. Broadening the scope of the inquiry, scholars have noted that traditional Arab rhetoric models several vital elements found in proverbs. For instance, the principles of concision (*'ijaz'*) and condensation (*'al-tawhid'*) have been valued for centuries by Arab rhetoricians (Al-Antiel, 1978; Al-Thaalibi, 1987, cited in Messir, 1984 and Al-Krenawi, 1998b, 1999).

Al-Krenawi (1999) made systematic therapeutic use of proverbs in his work with Bedouin-Arabs in both psychiatric outpatient and primary health care settings. The researcher noted that, compared to western patients, this population often appears not only disinclined, but also unable, to report their distress in psychological terms, thus resorting to somatic presentations. As against this view, Al-Krenawi attributed the largely somatic presentation of the Arab women to other factors, such as seeking help in a bio-medical setting. Further, as noted in the previous chapter, such help-seeking behavior by Arab/Muslim women in the Middle East may reflect a variety of cultural constraints (e.g., stigma, cultural management of female psychological distress). Finally, the above-discussed lack of cultural cleavage of soma and psyche in non-western cultures should be taken into account when considering these presentations.

In several chapters of this book we explore the mental and physical health challenges of the Arab women in the Middle East, and the ways in which cultural constructions impact on this theme. These concerns are evidenced in the language used by these women, and most vividly in the proverbs that they choose to express their state of distress. At this point we will examine several of these proverbs, which were first described in Al-Krenawi (1999, pp. 97-98).

A large number of Bedouin-Arab women are in polygamous relationships. We have reviewed in previous chapters the anguish for Islamic women associated with this marital structure: now we shall see how some woman formulated this suffering in proverbial terms. In a choice that spotlights the function of proverb as contradiction, one female patient uttered, *'Sa Asbor Hata Yjaz Al-Sabr An Sabri'* ('I will be patient until the patience gives up from my patience'). The husband of this patient had just entered into polygamy, recently taking a second wife. The tenor of the proverb was despair; the patient 'chose' patience, as no other strategy lay open to her. But the patience would inevitably leave her, and she would be left with her pain. A second patient exclaimed, *'Alain Baserah Walead Kaserah'* ('My eye is blind and my hand is short'). This woman's husband too had married another woman, and the proverb she chose expresses her belief – and that of her community - that an inability to satisfy her husband caused him to engage in polygamy. A third example is a typical one heard from first wives in polygamous families: *'Al-Darah Morah Lo Kanat Edan Jarah'* (The second wife is very sour, even if it is a handle of the pot'). This 'proverb of analogy' reflects the intense jealousy often found in this marital form, and the sentiment of first wives that subsequent wives are insignificant, as valueless as the handle of a pot.

Response to intimate partner violence was quite evident in the women's selection of proverbs. An abusive marital relationship was alluded to with the proverb *'Abnemshi Al-Hiatt Al-Hiatt Wa Benqual Ya rab Al-sotrah, Wamosh Mastorein'* ('I walk beside the wall and look for safety, but I am not safe'). That is, no matter how this patient attempted to 'blend in with the wall,' avoiding spousal conflict, she was unable to achieve her goal. Another victim of IPV stated *'Ale Ma Bedri Bequal yaa rath Fe Dearna'* ('strangers would say "I wish such a person were a member of my family"'). The patient chose this proverb for its ironic impact: her husband beat her.

Mirrored too, in the proverbs used by many Arab women living with marital discord was the sense of hopelessness and helplessness that we encountered in previous chapters dealing with the cultural management of women's mental health needs in the Arab region. A popular proverb with such patients was, *'Mn Baad Al-sabar Ila Al-Qabar'* ('After much patience and frustration, the situation will lead to the grave'). In a very harsh way, this example portrays the power of the proverb as 'equipment for living' (Whaley, 1993). That is, the speaker has resigned herself to a life of torment, ending only with death. This is not the life that we hope for, but it is the life that is lived by innumerable persons the world over. The Arab proverb chosen by this Bedouin-Arab patient reflects her effort to prepare herself for the life that she is currently living.

There was ample evidence in the proverbs of Arab women's reactions to 'honor'-based violence. The sibling of one patient, the sheikh of her tribe, had been murdered in 'honor'-code inter-tribal warfare. This patient expressed her grieving as she explained *'Johi Yaa Ean Wla tabhali Ala Ahiah'* ('Weep my eyes, and do not be shy for my brother'). The brother was described as *'Jamal Al-Asherah'* (the 'camel of the tribe', that is, the great provider, characterized by power and patience).

Finally, the phenomenon of arranged marriage was strongly reflected in the proverbs chosen by these patients. A male patient reported love for a woman from a different tribe, and the way in which the relationship was curtailed and proscribed by the woman's family and community. While anti-depressant medication was prescribed for this depressed young man, he found specific relief in his work with the social worker, during which he offered the proverb, *'Lawin winin al-Hoiar Yoma Albal Qutarath A'enah'* ('I will cry like the small camel when the other camels left him alone'). The patient was employing this proverb as a speech act.

Thus, it is clear that patients in the Arab region make prodigious use of proverbs to convey a range of feelings pertaining to their emotional states. In the view of Al-Krenawi (1999), these patients expect that the therapist will glean the gist of their affect from the proverb, enabling the patient to rely on such terse communication for getting across a sense of the individual's psychic dilemma. Notably, we have seen that these proverbs are exploited by Arab patients to bring to light responses to deeply painful conditions. These conditions constitute the cornerstone of the cultural scene in the Arab Middle East.

Conclusion

Proverbs have been characterized as 'medicine' (Burke, 1941, cited in Whaley, 1993). This healing function has been related to the way in which proverbs 'name' human distress, and the sense of relief that typically results from that act (Whaley, 1993). Proverbs, then, and metaphors, can function in the service of the amelioration of distress. In this chapter, we have wound the thread of somatic experience around a number of issues germane to the topic of Arab women's mental health in the Middle East. Specifically, we have seen how ethnic Vietnamese use of proverbs reveals a facility for psychological interpretation, and how the use of proverbs and metaphors by women in the Middle East uncovers a mother lode of emotional depth that 'constitute individual embodied expressions that are linked metaphorically to key conflicts at the interpersonal and societal level...' (Hinton & Lewis-Fernández, 2010, p. 4). In the next chapter, 'Diviners and Diagnosticians,' we consider another expression of key conflicts, the state of possession, and explore how this idiom of distress is manifested in the Arab region. At the same time, we will see how philosophies of living in this society drive this idiom, and how metaphor can be a crucial mechanism of treatment within it.

> 'Man is said to be a compound of soul and body. However proper this may be in religion, it is not so in medicine. He is, in the eye of a physician, a single and indivisible being, for so intimately united are his soul and body that one cannot be moved without the other. ' -- Benjamin Rush

Chapter 7
From Diviners to Diagnosticians: *Al-Junun*

Overview

Distress is always mediated. Nichter (2010) wrote 'of the role practitioners (from diagnosticians to diviners) play in framing experiences and expressions of distress in ways that Obeyesekere (1985, 1990) later came to refer to as the work of culture' (p. 401). In this chapter, we will delve into the ways in which this 'work of culture' manifests itself in the Arab world vis-à-vis emotional distress. We will begin with exploring how distress is configured in the Arab world, noting especially its traditional origins as something 'foreign' to the afflicted. Next, we will consider how traditional healers ('diviners') have worked within Arab culture to restore a sense of wellbeing to suffering individuals –and, critically in the case of Arab/Islamic society, to the community of such persons. Later on, we will turn to the biomedical tradition ('diagnosticians') and see how western psychotherapeutic assumptions and methods may run counter to enculturations in the Arab region. In this endeavor, we will recall Kirmayer & Young's admonition that, 'culturally mediated attitudes toward the body shape individuals' attention, interpretation and response to bodily symptoms, which in turn may aggravate or alleviate distress (1998, p.426). Thus, the somatic strain so well voiced by the Arab women we encountered in the previous chapters will be heard plainly, a refrain that resounds again and again in the Arab region.

Al-Junun

'Junun' is the Arabic word for insanity, and its root is the word 'jinn'; that is, 'demon.' This term has been traced to the Qur'an, as well as to Aramaic, the latter implying a pre-Islamic origin (Al-Ashquar, 2005; Albright, 1940, cited in Lim, Hoek & Blom, 2014). The derivation reflects the fact that in traditional Arab culture, the source of emotional distress is understood to be external to the suffering individual, and typically caused by some sort of possessing force. This force may control the thoughts, desires and actions of the patient. However, despite this fundamental etiological externalization, there exists a sense that within the social orbit of the sufferer one may discern problems that precipitated the distress: female jealousy, for example, might be harnessed through the powers of a witch, the evil eye, or potions to debilitate the object of the antagonism (Dwairy, 1998; Al-Issa, 2000).

Jinn Belief in Contemporary Islamic Society

Lim et al. (2014) surveyed the biomedical literature on jinn belief in an effort to identify topics that were pertinent to mental health services. They found that, 'the belief in jinn continues to be deeply embedded in everyday life in many Islamic communities' (p. 4). This conviction is not exclusive to Islamic communities in the Arab region. Indeed, recent surveys conducted by a number of scholars confirm that Muslims throughout the United Kingdom and Bangladesh ascribe to the notion of jinn and related concepts (Mullick, Khalifa, Nahar, & Walker, 2013; Khalifa, Hardie, Latif, Jamil & Walker, 2011). Notably, the denial of the existence of jinn may result in a Moslem person being labeled *kaafir,* that is, a non-believer (Ameen, 2005, cited in Lim et al., 2014).

Concerns of heresy also play a prominent role in the silence that reigns, especially in non-Islamic settings, with regard to discussion of jinn-related topics. The broaching of such subjects may leave Muslims apprehensive that they will be considered unfaithful to the dictates of the Qur'an (Lim, et al., 2014). Too, anxiety exists about 'bringing on' the jinn through their mention (Drieskens, 2008, cited in Lim et al., 2014). Finally, fears of being ostracized figure into the question. While jinn belief is part and parcel of Islamic life even today, it is not without its negative connotations. That is to say, while considered among Muslims a natural and expectable aspect of the human condition, jinn involvement, with its associations of mental illness, is a highly loaded issue.

Islam and Locus of Control

The Islamic notion of the 'will of Allah' also intensively informs the Arab view of mental illness (Dwairy, 1998). As this factor is also external to the suffering individual him or herself, this notion may serve to reduce perceived responsibility for one's fate (see Rai's final comment above). The locus of control is positioned outside of the individual, in accordance with the authoritarian lifestyle that typifies this region.

El-Islam (1998) highlighted this cultural externalization of locus of control when he wrote that, 'native healers fit the general cultural tendency toward projection rather than personal responsibility' (cited in Dwairy, 1998, p. 120). In line with this notion, in Dwairy's view, ethnic Arabs are disinclined to seek out psychotherapy because they do not ascribe to the belief that individual or interpersonal conflict is related to emotional distress. Help at times of distress is sought, instead, from the biomedical system or from traditional healers. Indeed, the view that medical doctors, native healers, religious leaders or family members (as against mental health professionals) are the correct avenue for those seeking help for emotional distress is quite diffused in the Arab world (Okasha et al., 1994; Timimi, 1995, cited in Dwairy, 1998).

Traditional Arab-Region Treatments

Traditional treatment is understood to counter the effects of a malevolent force (the 'jinn') external to the patient. A popular example of such treatment is the *zar* ceremony. This ceremony is an Arab-region healing ritual that accords with traditional Arab views on the proper response to personal distress. In this group-oriented ceremony, the possession of the afflicted individual is identified and managed through contact between the foreign entity and the sufferer (Al-Sabai, 1989, cited in Dwairy, 1998). A variety of vocal, instrumental and movement techniques are used to precipitate a trance state for the participants, who are then free to verbalize otherwise prohibited desires and concerns. Recalling our exploration of metaphor and its work in chapter five, this trance state, according to Kirmayer (2004):

> ...is a metaphor for states of absorption, concentration, distraction, or 'awayness' in which attention is turned inward or away from ordinary consensual external reality... it reflects scripted social behavior that unfolds according to the dramatic requirements of stage, setting and dialogue. Healing

> practices that are designed to carry the healer, the patient or the audience into an absorbed or trance-like state, both mark off the event as special and allow participants to focus on images that can be worked on through the sensory, emotional and imaginative processes evoked by metaphor. The ritual use of trance then has more to do with specific meaning conveyed by the context and metaphors of healing than with any generic change in state (Kirmayer, 2004, pp. 40-41).

In the context of the *zar* ceremony, 'ordinary, consensual external reality' is constituted by the confines of the highly ordered, rigidly hierarchical Arab society; the 'scripted social behavior that unfolds according to the dramatic requirements' are the dance and song of the practice; the 'event being marked off as special' is the contact with the intrusive, harmful force, and the 'specific meaning conveyed by the context' is the acknowledgement of illicit thoughts and feelings, emanating from the patient but attributed to a spirit. When the spirit is duly appeased, sometimes through animal sacrifice, the hoped-for 'change in state' can be one of relief and positive mood, which in turn may have 'significant effects on autonomic, endocrine and immune functioning with consequences for healing, health and well-being' (Kirmayer, 2004, p. 41).

Conceptually consonant with the evil eye or jinn notions, the *zar* ritual locates the locus of control outside the person in distress. This is echoed by Dwairy (1998) in his description of the ceremony as a kind of cathartic outlet for the drives given no other permissible space by authoritarian Arab society. Homeostasis, too, is achieved, and the community, so quintessentially central to Arab life, is maintained in balance. As Kirmayer (2004) has put it:

> the healing practice is conducted in a way that its performance already implies a kind of closure, completeness and success...symbolically, at least, everything has been restored to its proper place (Kirmayer, 2004, p. 43).

Another traditional healing ritual, performed both in public and private venues, is the exorcism. This is a ritual common to multiple Arab countries. As in the *zar* ritual, the healer and spirit engage in dialogue, and the healer, through a variety of possible means (adjuration, threat, corporeal, sacrificial) aims to expel the noxious spirit (Dwairy, 1998). Here, too, the elements of external locus of control, projection and active clinical stance are well illustrated in an early report on the fusion of traditional and biomedical treatments. In his investigation of dervish treatment among Bedouin-Arabs in the Negev, Al-Krenawi (1998b) noted that the traditional healer took a highly active role in the typically public treatment of his patients. The latter, in contrast, remained quite passive in the course of the vigorous treatment:

> ...the Dervishes rarely asked questions of the patients. Instead, after ascertaining the cause of their illness by looking at their symptoms, touching their heads, or examining some item belonging to the patient, they would proceed to energetically expel the evil spirits. They would communicate, sometimes loudly and angrily, with the spirits, and give the patient instructions. Sometimes they would even beat the spirits out of the patients. Throughout it all, the patients remained passive...the healers took pains to assure the patients that their illness wasn't of their own making but something that came upon them from outside, whether directly from God or evil spirits or through the agency of sorcery or the evil eye. Being able to project their problem left the patients feeling good about themselves and strengthened their determination to fight the illness...the healers and their patients share the same 'poetic' terminology of illness...(Al-Krenawi, 1998b, p. 14).

Here we may highlight an important point, noted as something of an aside in the above-provided description of dervish work. The author informs us that in the context of traditional healing, the client and the clinician share a *poetic terminology of illness*. We have spoken throughout this volume about the poetics of illness expression. We have seen how it has been described as an idiom of distress, and, most relevantly for women in the Arab region, a somatic idiom of distress. We have noted how these poetics have taken the form of proverbs, of metaphors and, mostly literally, of song itself. In his piece on Celan's poetry of alterity, Kirmayer (2007) wrote of how such an approach can enrich the clinical experience of East and West alike:

> ...I have tried to show some ways in which languages of suffering involve metaphoric constructions that are often fragmentary, tentative, and contradictory. Understanding and responding to this language demands a poetics of illness experience... While the halting efforts of patients to articulate their experience in clinical settings usually do not involve the same self-conscious efforts at refinement and concision that allow the poet to fashion the poem as an esthetic object, they use some of the same faculties of imagination to try to reach the other and call forth an empathetic and healing response (Kirmayer, 2007, pp. 20-21).

In several chapters of this book we read of the ways in which Bedouin-Arab women exercise these 'same faculties of imagination.' Their 'calling forth of a healing response' may yet be answered, both on an individual and communal level. In the next chapter, we will discuss how our findings may constitute a cornerstone for a new kind of structure, one that is specifically designed to cater to the mental health needs of women in the Arab world.

In all these traditional Arab-region rituals, the traditional practitioner takes a highly directive stance. This is in line with the expectations of traditional Arab society, in which the healer is viewed as an authority figure, a '*hakim*' (wise individual) (Al-Krenawi & Graham, 1996a; West, 1987, cited in Al-Krenawi & Graham, 1999). This perspective mirrors the authoritarian, hierarchical structure of Arab society, and is evident as well in the way in which ethnic Arab patients relate to the biomedical system. Indeed, Al-Krenawi and Graham (1999) partially explain their patients' inability to name their psychiatric diagnoses by noting that the patients felt that they did not need to so engage with their treatment, as they were already in the hands of a responsible medical professional.

In the Arab world, neither jinn *belief* nor traditional healing *actions* are relics of the Arab/Islamic past. States in the Arab region have made singularly unsuccessful juridical attempts to ban such treatments. As with many culturally embedded behaviors (polygamy for example, as discussed earlier) legislation has proven to be a fairly flimsy tool. Despite the fact that a number of countries in the Arab region have outlawed the use of these methods (Al-Issa, 2000), patients in the Arab world resort to traditional healing on a very large scale. They are so ingrained in the region that only recently Beeble et al. (2009) reported that in the UAE nearly one-half of psychiatric patients had pursued non-professional treatment before turning to psychiatry for help. Some Arab patients seek traditional assistance alongside biomedical help, and a limited overlap in the treatment systems has been reported. In fact, nearly, four decades ago, Racy (1980) noted that, 'Native social workers therefore can become, and occasionally have been used as, important agents of change' (p. 215). Thus far, however, this prediction has not been borne out. Recently, Okasha et al. (2012) found an overall dearth of interaction between traditional healers and medical practitioners in the region (cited in Sewilam, 2014). In the next chapter, we will return to this issue, and there present preliminary thoughts on how Racy's early call for traditional/biomedical interpenetration in the treatment of women in the Arab region may be answered by a novel project that is rooted in the findings of the research presented in chapter seven.

Ethnic Arab self-narratives in psychotherapy

It has been made clear that, 'calling attention to the body in pain or discomfort is one way to let others know something is wrong' (Kirmayer, 1984, p. 159). In psychological venues as well as primary care biomedical ones, patients in the Arab region have been found to focus initially on their somatic complaints and avoid direct discussion of their feelings and moods (Al-Issa, 1995; Al-Krenawi, 1999a, 1999b, 1998; El-Islam, 1994, 1975, cited in Al-Krenawi, 2002). However, the picture is not unidimensional, even at this juncture. While presenting initially rosy views of their family life, ethnic Arabs also use metaphoric language, as discussed throughout this volume, to allude to emotional distress. The simile-driven phrase 'my heart feels like a dark room'(Bazzoui, 1970; Timimi, 1995, cited in Dwairy, 1998, p. 124) is quite a pointed reference to psychological pain, in spite of its body-directed semantics. Later in this chapter, we will explore some clinical avenues for work with metaphor.

Language and Locus of Control

The top-down structure of Arab society is well reflected in the expectations of Arab patients in the Islamic region. As locus of control for illness is located from without the patient, so too is locus of control for wellness externally located. In other words, in as much as the Arab cultural environment disinclines the Arab patient to attribute emotional distress to his or her own intrapsychic or interpersonal conflicts, it also inhibits the development of assuming responsibility for personal change. The hoped-for change is expected to emerge from the conduct of the clinician. West put it baldly: 'The concept of working to improve the self is generally nonexistent in Arab cultures' (West, 1987, cited in Dwairy, 1998, p. 124).

As the primary mode of 'talk therapy' is speech, any evaluation of its perception among a group must be done within the context of a given culture's use of language. In Arab cultures, talking is primarily used to 'give directives…or to express those feelings that are acceptable but not necessarily authentic' (Dwairy, 1998, p. 140). Hence, ethnic Arab patients do not have a frame that encompasses the bedrock of psychodynamic psychotherapy; that is, that talk can be used to achieve insight-driven personal change. Instead, they come to the therapist with an expectation similar to that which they hold of the biomedical physician (or the traditional healer): that they will receive something from the authority figure that will put an end to their distress. Even psychiatrists are not expected to engage the patient in any form of talk therapy: examinations and medicine are the expected clinical response (Al-Krenawi and Graham, 1999a; Al-Krenawi et al., 2000;

Ibrahim and Ibrahim, 1993, cited in Al-Krenawi, 2002). In the case of the physician, the Arab patient tends to expect to receive medication (according to Racy (1980), large, colorful pills are considered best); in the case of the psychotherapist, the Arab patient tends to expect to receive directive advice.

Divergence in Philosophies of Living

The divergence in tone and tenor between Arab region and western clinical encounters can be partially attributed to the different philosophies of proper living that drive the two groups. Many thought leaders in the field of developmental psychology have emphasized the concepts of individuation and separation from the family of origin (Erikson, 1993; Mahler, 1968; Mahler, Bergman, and Pine, 1995, cited in Dwairy, 1998). In the western world, persons who do not follow this trajectory are considered to be abnormal. The western psychotherapeutic thrust has been to assist the individual in getting on with these culturally valorized tasks.

By way of contrast, traditional Arab culture decidedly *devalues* these notions. Instead, as discussed in previous chapters, Arab society esteems the group as a whole, with the individual considered only a part of the critical collective. Identity is gained – and sustained – through group membership. Age does not fundamentally alter this cultural fact: adults and children alike are expected to remain within a highly interdependent web of familial and tribal relationships. Behavior contrary to this norm is considered deviant, and worthy of punishment (Dwairy, 1992a, 1992b, 1992c, cited in Dwairy, 1998).

One Size Does Not Fit All: Western Methods in the Arab Region

Dwairy (1998) clarifies how a wide range of western psychotherapeutic techniques, each in its own way, can run counter to the enculturation of ethnic Arab persons. For instance, the impulses that emerge in the course of psychodynamic treatment are both prohibited in Arab culture, and, when expressed, engender conflict between the patient and his or her family. The 'true self' that emerges in humanistic therapy may collide with the dictates of the community in which the ethnic Arab patient lives. Cognitively-based training may imbue the patient with a 'logic' that militates against that taught by his or her collective environment. The 'democratic balance' encouraged by western family systems therapies may threaten to topple the inflexible hierarchical structure of the family in the Middle East. Thus:

> … the promotion of self-efficacy, self-expression, and self-actualization… engenders external conflicts with which clients are not prepared to cope. Rather than alleviating internal, intrapsychic conflicts, this treatment approach will likely result in a great deal of societal and familial conflict for clients…Gaining awareness of personal wishes that cannot be met in their society will only lead to greater frustration, helplessness, and anger, which will not help reduce psychological problems…This environmental conflict is iatrogenic in that the problems originated from the treatment itself (Dwairy and Van Sickle, 1996; Dwairy, 1998, p. 138).

Along these lines, Kirmayer and Young (1998) affirm that:

> …the introduction of psychological language as a way of understanding a problem is also introducing a culture-specific concept of the person, which may conflict with the values…of the culture of origin and so create new dilemmas… (Kirmayer & Young, 1998, p. 427).

These 'new dilemmas' have deep consequences. Scholars have reported the adverse effects of attempts to 'empower' women in the Arab region. Racy (1980) found that 'Encouragement of the woman's autonomy or self-assertion is likely to engender trouble' (p. 214). And Dwairy (1998) noted multiple cases in which patients were 'helped' to uncover unconscious wishes that were related to the presenting symptoms, only to be left in a depressed state when their attempts to reconcile their newly revealed desires with their environments failed. As the author wryly wrote, 'the operation was successful, but [the patient] was left with an open wound' (Dwairy, 1998, p. 182).

Of course, we are not dealing with an either/or situation. Conceptual overlaps do exist. Like western humanists, Islamic patients in the Arab region also know of a personal 'true self.' However, the parameters of this self-identity differ quite markedly from that of the humanistic-oriented person. The Koran teaches that 'a life without faith is a state of spiritual non-being in which one loses touch with his/her true self' (Koran, Surah 49, v. 19, cited in Al-Krenawi & Graham, 1999). Thus, from the point of view of an Islamic Arab patient, the realization of one's true self is contingent upon the success of achieving two superordinate goals: correct relationship with the Divine (Allah) and correct relationship with the community.

In his recent work on transcultural psychiatry and globalization,

Kirmayer (2006) reminds us that:

> To penetrate the psychological depths of the person...one must look not only inside the individual but at the social contexts in which they live, at their developmental trajectory, and the communities, both local and distant, in which they participate (p.132).

This is the point at which one may profitably consider intervention in the Arab communities in the Middle East. This region, then, presents a specific and complex therapeutic challenge. As everywhere, clinicians in the Arab region are called upon to treat suffering individuals without introducing unproductive iatrogenic distress. Here, however, avoiding such an outcome hinges on the clinician having a deep understanding of the embeddedness of the individual in his/her community, of the enculturated perception of (external) locus of control, and of the somatic orientation of illness expression. In the next section of this chapter, we will turn to several possibilities for achieving such successful clinical outcomes.

Metaphor Therapies

As demonstrated above, women in the Arab region frequently recur to somatic metaphoric language in their expression of distress. Thus, one natural point of entry for psychotherapeutic treatment of this population is metaphor therapy. Erickson (1935; 1944) and Kopp (1971, 1972) pioneered work in this field (Witztum, van der Hart and Friedman,1988). Orthony, Reynolds, and Alter (1978) explain that, 'Although metaphors occur...at the level of individual sentences the really crucial role they play is in systems. We may call them extended metaphors or analogies, or even metaphorical models' (Witztum et al., 1988, p.1). These, as well as individual metaphoric sentences such as metaphoric kernel statements (Fernandez, 1977) are common in psychotherapy (Witztum et al., 1988). With regard to therapeutic efficacy, Witztum et al. tell us:

> ...metaphors make the language more poetic and picturesque. The relevance for psychotherapy is that language can be examined as an index of the natural imagistic content of a patient's thinking. This provides the clinician with a point of departure for joining with the patient during treatment (Witztum, 1988, p. 2).

In the previous chapter, we discussed the cultural expectation in the

Arab region that helping persons will be the active force in the therapeutic encounter. This is not exclusive to the Islamic world. Witztum et al. (1988) note that in western psychotherapy as well, the creative force often initially comes from the therapist. While acknowledging that using metaphors to share an experience is quite creative, these researchers contend that patients suffer from a kind of 'frozen metaphorization' by which their true creativity is stymied. In their view, the job of the clinician is to 'unthaw the patient's creative energy and propel it into problem-solving activities' (Witztum et al., 1988, p. 2).

Along somewhat different lines, Dwairy (1998) reviews three types of metaphor therapies: Ericksonian interventions, Knopp's metaphor therapy, and Bresler's Drawing of the Problem and Solution treatment (p. 171-172). These will be outlined below, followed by a construction of how each models might be applied to the metaphor-based treatment of Arab/Islamic women.

Noting that Erickson employed metaphor in the service of both diagnosis and treatment, Dwairy (1998, p. 170) highlighted Erickson's use of the notion of 'utilization,' that is, a 'strategic response' to what the client brings into the treatment. For instance, the 'stone-like sensation' described by the patient of one of Erickson's colleagues was taken up by the therapist in a concrete healing ritual that involved the fusing of metaphor and psychic pain (Zeig, 1995, cited in Dwairy, p. 171). Al-Krenawi (1998) described such a fusion in his work with grieving Arab-Bedouin widows. In that context, the therapist made use of the traditional Arab mourning meal, known as '*rahmana*,' to treat his clients' survivor-based fears of retaliation.

Kopp's metaphor therapy entails four phases: (1) Identification of client-introduced metaphor(s); (2) Client elaboration of problem through metaphor; (3) Client pursuance of solution within the context of the metaphor; and (4) Client application of metaphoric solution to the problem at hand (Kopp, 1995 cited in Dwairy, 1998). Al-Krenawi's (2014) work with polygamous families provides an example of the way in which this technique might be applied with women in the Arab region. As we have seen in chapter five, Arab women whose husbands enter into polygamy speak of their plight in richly metaphoric language. While the management of feelings around actual death was discussed in the previous paragraph on Ericksonian treatment, the engagement of affect around metaphoric death is at issue in this instance. That is to say, Bedouin-Arab senior wives have been reported to portray their sense of loss around polygamy in metaphoric terms such as: 'For me, he [the husband] is dead' (Al-Krenawi, Graham and Salem, 1997, p. 454). Nonetheless, these researchers found that they were able to engage the multiple wives as well as the husband in polygamous families around carefully chosen issues, such as the mutual benefit of their children's interests. Thus, beginning where the female Arab client is, in this case with the metaphor of death around engagement in polygamy, the therapist might use Kopp's method to help her client arrive at a metaphor-driven, vital solution that, while directly benefiting her children, will improve concomitantly her sense of self. This is, of course, only one of many typical themes for the Arab female patient, and Kopp's technique is amenable for use with the full gamut of solution-oriented work with women in the Arab region.

Taking another tack, Bresler's (1994) metaphor-based treatment emphasizes pain management. This technique, termed by Bresler, 'mind-controlled analgesia,' is doubly useful in the Arab region (Bresler,1994, cited in Dwairy, 1998, p. 173). In the treatment regimen, the patient sketches three pictures. Picture number one is to depict 'pain,' picture number two, 'pain at its best,' and picture number three, something pleasurable. The patient is instructed to manipulate in her mind's eye the metaphoric images, thus achieving pain toleration. As here we are confronted with a complex mix of physical and emotional pain, Bresler's technique offers a dual opportunity to assist Arab/Islamic female patients. We have read above of the emotional detritus of living with the threat of polygamy, 'honor-based' violence, and other patriarchal cultural practices, and we have learned of the somatic expression to which Arab/Islamic female patients are inclined. While the therapist lacks the ability to divest her patients' lives of pain, she may be able to use what Dwairy (1998, p. 173) refers to as intervention 'in the metaphoric-imaginative realm' to help them tolerate the pain associated with those realities. Indeed, toleration of (at least temporarily) unavoidable pain is the cornerstone of the next modality, mindfulness treatment.

Mindfulness Treatment

The term *mindfulness* derives from the Pali word *sati*, which encompasses the actions of awareness, attention and remembering (Bodhi, 2000, cited in Davis & Hayes, 2011). It has been proposed that mindfulness be defined pragmatically as 'moment-to-moment awareness of one's experience without judgment' (Davis & Hayes, 2011, p. 198).

Mindfulness has attracted a great deal of academic (as well as popular) interest in the past several decades (Didonna, 2009; Shapiro & Carlson, 2009, cited in Davis & Hayes, 2011). The literature points to the notion that mindfulness training may 'elicit positive emotions, minimize negative affect and rumination and enable effective emotional regulation' (Davis & Hayes, 2011, p. 200). With regard to the treatment of anxiety and depression among women in the Arab region, mindfulness-based therapy has been found to be effective in reducing symptoms of these disorders. For instance, in Hofman, S.G., Sawyer, Witt, and Oh's 2010 meta-analysis of 39 studies in which Mindfulness-Based Stress Reduction (MBSR) and mindfulness-based cognitive therapy formed the bulk of the therapies, a large effect size was found among clinical populations suffering from anxiety and depression, and a moderate effect size was found among non-clinical populations (cited in Davis & Hayes, 2011). In the nineteen studies that involved long-term follow-up of anxiety and depressive symptoms, moderate effect sizes were found. Broadening the picture, Hoffman et al. (2010) put forth that the processes that underlie multiple clinical problems may be positively affected by mindfulness-based treatments (Davis & Hayes, 2011). As such, it is reasonable to explore whether this treatment is indicated for the somatization behaviors found to be prevalent among women in the Arab region.

A small but growing body of research has investigated the effects of mindfulness therapy on somatization disorder and functional somatic syndromes. As long-term follow-up and control groups are lacking in the literature on mindfulness therapies, Overby Fjorback, Arendt, Ornbol, Walach, Rehfeld, Schroder, and Fink's (2012) randomized trial with one-year follow-up represents an important addition to the body of knowledge. These researchers found that among the 119 patients randomly assigned to mindfulness treatment or enhanced treatment-as-usual (two-hour specialist medical treatment and brief cognitive therapy), more rapid improvement was found following mindfulness therapy than enhanced treatment-as-usual.

As mindfulness is frequently taught in the context of a short-term (eight-week) session program, and is highly goal-oriented as well as directive in nature, it accords quite well with the recommendations for treatment of Arab/Islamic women found in the literature. Nonetheless, as they typically involve individual intervention, metaphor therapies and mindfulness training lack the most crucial component of work among this population: family involvement. Hence, in the following section, we will turn to what is perhaps the preeminent modality for Arab/Islamic communities in general and Arab/Islamic women in particular: family therapy.

Family Treatment

In the highly sociocentric (see chapter 2) Arab culture, 'systems of healing typically involve rituals that engage the whole family, clan, or community. The healing intervention thus affirms the person's connectedness and aims to repair or reorder relationships with others' (Adponle, Whitley and Kirmayer, 2012 p. 118). While this principle is strikingly evident in the community healing *zar* ritual, described in the previous chapter, as we will see below, it can be exploited in the biomedical arena by the culturally sensitive use of family treatment.

Due to the highly interdependent nature of life in Arab societies, family work may be considered the heart of treatment in the Arab region. Importantly, this is true even for patients who present on an individual basis, and especially so for the female patient. Strict attention, however, must be paid to the social structure of the family and community. Dwairy (1998) has cautioned that, 'Solutions should be sought within the cultural field of the family' (p. 166). As the cultural field of the Arab family is patriarchal and hierarchal, the family authority figure, typically the father, must be made to feel that the treatment will not detract in any way from his status. In Dwairy's view, 'creating a safe environment for the authority is a necessary precondition for successful therapy with traditional families' (Dwairy, 1998, p. 166). This project of developing a safe environment for the authority can be accomplished in a number of ways. One element is the *eco-map*, described below.

Eco-maps have proven exceptionally helpful in the treatment of the Arab family. Developed in the 1970s by sociologist Ann Hartman, this tool is 'a graphic representation or visualization of the family and linkages to the larger social system including informal (e.g., friends, extended family members) and formal (e.g., early care and education providers, early intervention providers) supports' (McCormick, Stricklin, Nowak & Rous, 2008, p. 1). Based on Urie Bronfenbrenner's (1979) ecological model of human development, the eco-map literally maps out the interwovenness of the family system.

In his work among both monogamous and polygamous Arab-Bedouin, Al-Krenawi (1997, 1998, 2001, 2014) has shown that successful family intervention with these populations rests on the ability of the clinician to read the eco-map of the family and sub-families. Further, and in line with Dwairy (1998) noted above, the author has argued, 'that change is most successfully implemented with the active participation of the father, recognizing his considerable power over...subfamily systems' (Al-Krenawi,

1997, p. 455). Interestingly, however, while in traditional Arab families (both monogamous and polygamous) change cannot take place without the involvement of the father, the 'change-instigator' may be a different figure entirely. In Al-Krenawi (2014), we learn of an exceptionally large and complex multi-unit polygamous family in which the four co-wives and sixty children were in marked and ongoing distress. The author/therapist there described significant, positive and family-wide change that was initiated by none other than the fourth and youngest wife. Of course, a great deal of preparatory work had to be done by the clinician before this change could be set into motion. This work centered on the two points thus far emphasized in this section: the construction of a clear space of safety and respect for the father, and the careful selection of a target system for intervention. In that context, when the father experienced his status as secure, he acted with a certain degree of openness to altering his behavior. It is crucial to note here the manner in which the father was approached by the clinician. The intervention was framed as an opportunity for the father to better fulfill his paternal obligations as the head of a large family that looked to him for support and guidance. In this way, the hierarchal, patriarchal configuration was left totally intact. Too, when the target system chosen was the improved functioning of the children, rather than, say, directly fulfilling the needs of one or another of the wives (an unacceptable goal in this cultural field), the eco-map was interpreted with cultural competence. Hence, powered by the dual engines of respect for family structure and culturally competent choice of intervention target, family treatment reveals itself to be the treatment of choice in the Arab family system. The research presented in the next chapter provides further insight into how the somatic idioms of distress used by Bedouin Arab women, both of Western Egypt and of the Negev, are expressed in their lived experiences.

Z'ama ya l-yas iz-zol...
Willa rafig dima lkhatri...

I wonder, is despair
A phantom or my companion for life...

-- Alwad 'Ali Bedouin poem, from Abu-Lughod, *Veiled Sentiments*

Chapter 8
Women of Somatic Metaphor: Bedouin Arab Women of the Negev

The honor and modesty codes that serve as fundaments to Arab societies have been explored in previous chapters. As well, we have seen how women in these communities often resort to the poetic devices of metaphor and proverb to express what is otherwise culturally unacceptable to convey. In this chapter, we will deepen the discussion in two ways. First, we see how these codes have been managed and manipulated by the poetic use of language among women of the Awlad 'Ali Bedouin community in Western Egypt; second, we will learn how the cultural cousins of the Awlad 'Ali, the Bedouin of southern Israel, used somatic language to express loneliness and longing in an investigation of the use of one primary care facility in the region

Metaphor: A Form of Poetry

In *Veiled Sentiments*, Lila Abu-Lughhod's study of *ghinnawa* ('little songs'; traditional poetry sung mostly by women to women) among the Awlad 'Ali Bedouin in western Egypt, we are told a striking thing: the Awlad 'Ali women use *ghinnawa* to 'express sentiments that violate the very moral code they uphold so passionately with their practice of modesty' (1999, p. xxi). In the same context, however, Abu-Lughod carefully noted that the 'defiance of or resistance to [patriarchy]' suggested by authors such as Gloria Raheja and Ann Gold in describing the poems of Hindu women in North India is not found among the Awlad 'Ali women; that is, while the *ghinnawa* of the former defy the moral codes of honor and modesty, these women remain committed to those very codes (p. 1999, xxi-xxii). Further, and germane to our overall assessment of women's mental health in the Middle East, Abu-Luhghod wrote that in the polygamous Awlad 'Ali households she studied, poetry constituted the core – and sometimes sole – way in which feelings of jealousy and betrayal felt by co-wives could be expressed. In point of fact, after twenty years of anthropological fieldwork with the Awlad

'Ali the author was so struck by this notion that she made the following far-reaching claim regarding poetry and enculturation:

> These cases confirm the strong link between poetry and matters of love, romantic or conjugal, and justify us in designating the *ghinnswa* as a discourse of love. This discourse seems to be opposed to the mundane discourse of ordinary language structured by overt social values and honor-linked personal ideals. Individuals whose ordinary actions and statements conform to the modesty code, who take pains to present themselves as moral and worthy of respect, use poetry to comment on their personal fortunes and tribulations in love *and to express sentiments that violate the canons of modesty* (Abu-Lughod, 1999, p. 232, emphasis added).

This use of metaphor at the margins; that is, spoken by the least powerful, most dependent individuals in Awlad 'Ali society is hauntingly reminiscent of the metaphoric poetry spoken by their cultural kin, the Bedouin Arab women of the Negev. In Chapter 6, we saw how these women wield proverbs and metaphors to convey their anguish about the honor codes and polygamous marital structures that form the fulcrum of their society. Abu-Lughod ends her work with the thought:

> ...Awlad 'Ali's poetry of self and sentiment [may] be viewed as their corrective to an obsession with morality and an overzealous adherence to the ideology of honor. ...Poetry reminds people of another way of being...And maybe the vision is cherished because people sense that the costs of this system, in the limits it places on human experience, are just too high (Abu-Lughod, 1999, p. 259).

As we have seen, this 'obsession with morality' and 'overzealous adherence to the ideology of honor' is by no means unique to the Awlad 'Ali Bedouin of western Egypt, nor, in fact, to the Negev Bedouin of southern Israel. It is endemic to all patriarchal societies (recall India and China), and the Arab region is another location in which this worldview is expressed. Nonetheless, though these sentiments may be salient throughout much of the world, in this work we concentrate on the ways in which they impact on the mental health of Arab/Islamic women in the Middle East.

The themes of the *ghinnawas* are telling. Poems of despair predominate, with another distinct set drawing on the:

> ...imagery of bodily ills. Withering of the body, wasting away, dizziness, headaches, and unspecified pain are some of the poetic symptoms of painful emotional experiences... (Abu-Lughod, 1999, p. 270).

The themes of despair and enervation are highly imbricated: one feeds upon the other. The Bedouin women of both the Awad 'Ali and the Negev share these narratives, perhaps 'singing' them in different ways. Below, we turn to a brief sketch of Bedouin life in southern Israel, as well as an analysis of a large-scale study done by Al-Krenawi & Graham (2004) in which they explore the somatic symptom reporting of women in this population.

The Bedouin-Arabs of the Negev

Bedouin-Arab is a general term for the nomadic tribes of the Middle East and North Africa that originate from the Arabian Desert (Barakat, 1993). The Negev Bedouin constitute an enclave in Israel, and are distinct from, although related to, Bedouin communities in other countries. This is a traditional and conservative Middle Eastern community that functions within a modern state. Traditionally, the Bedouin-Arab, who are Muslim, were a nomadic people, but today they are undergoing a rapid and dramatic process of transition and change caused by sedentarization, urbanization and the influences of modernization (Al-Krenawi, 2013).

Bedouin-Arab society shares many social and cultural features of the wider Arab world. For instance, it is high-context and authoritarian (Hall, 1976; Barakat, 1993; Al-Krenawi, 2014). Bedouin-Arabs, like other Arab persons, are sociocentric, and thus link their identity with the collective identity of the family, the extended family and the tribe (Adeponle et al., 2012; Al-Krenawi, 2014). So, too, does Bedouin-Arab society subordinate its female to its male members. As we have reviewed in the chapters above, the family is hierarchically structured such that men are empowered over women and elders are empowered over youth (Mernissi, 1975; Abu-Lughod, 1986). Like elsewhere in the Arab region, the Bedouin-Arab culture is resoundingly patriarchal. Girls are expected to marry and bear children, male children in particular. Bedouin-Arab wives are expected to be present in their homes at all times, except when carrying out daily chores that take them out of the home (Mass & Al-Krenawi, 1994). Bedouin communities, like their non-Bedouin Arab kin, valorize family associations, family/female honor, and male progeny (Al-Sadawi, 1985; Shalhoub-Kevorkian, 1997; Al-Krenawi & Graham, 2014).

Bedouin-Arab culture mirrors the general Arab views on femininity and seduction, as well as lines of activity and passivity. In this frame, men are expected to behave in a traditionally 'active' manner, and women to act in a traditionally 'passive' one. Further, the notion that women are capable of surreptitiously controlling men with esoteric female wisdom is quite pervasive (Al-Krenawi, 2013; Mernissi, 1975). This view can be discerned as well in core Islamic texts (*Koran, Sura Yusuf,* V. 25-30). We now turn to a study that reveals some ways in which Bedouin-Arab women express their responses to the demands and constraints of their community. Later, in chapter eight, we will discuss the results of this study and consider how it can constitute the core of a plan for mental health intervention among Arab women in the Middle East.

Population

Approximately 220,000 Bedouin live in the Negev, which encompasses about one- third of the population in the region. Sixty thousand Bedouin live in the Galilee and nearly 10,000 in central Israel. The Negev Bedouin have the highest reproduction rate in Israel, approximately 3.5% in 2013. On average, families consist of 6.5 children (Inter-Israeli Task Force on Israeli Arab Issues, 2014, p. 1). Continuing at this rate, the Bedouin population would double every nineteen years. The Israel Land Administration anticipates that the Negev Bedouin population will reach 300,000 by the year 2020 (Inter-Israeli Task Force on Israeli Arab Issues, 2014, p. 1).

Economics

Animal husbandry was for millennia the stock-in-trade of nomadic societies. With the modern modification of the nomadic lifestyle, Bedouin communities throughout the Middle East have become more agriculturally oriented. Their share of market exchange in the region has also expanded, the commerce controlled by the communities' male members.

Like their sisters worldwide, Bedouin women for centuries carried out myriad and multifarious jobs, ranging from household and maternal chores to caring for the livestock, weaving, and producing dairy products. Traditionally, Bedouin men were responsible for the once-critical activities pertaining to inter-tribal relations, including both hosting guests and physical defense. With the sedentarization demanded by modernity and a consequent passing of those tasks, men in the Bedouin communities took on the role of political brokers between tribes and the surrounding states

(Beck and Keddie, 1978; Al-Krenawi, 2013). As well, Bedouin men have developed businesses that cater to the wider surrounding environment, such as trucking transportation services (Al-Krenawi, 2013). The tasks of Bedouin women have also changed with modernization, resulting, in the reckoning of scholars such as Abu-Rabia-Queder (2007), in a reduction in social status and personal perceptions of worth.

The Negev Bedouin rank highest in terms of disadvantaged communities in the state of Israel. This takes into account levels of poverty, unemployment and income. However, this society is undergoing a process of enhanced education and economic development. While the socio-economic gaps are still massive, there is an increasing number of Bedouin academics, businesspeople and civil society activists (Inter-Israeli Task Force, p. 1). Bedouin women particularly are spearheading this social advancement. Some of these points will be touched upon below.

Educational strides in the Bedouin-Arab community

One of the most far-reaching changes – or, more precisely, transformations – to take place among the Bedouin in Israel involves the education of its children in general, and the higher education of its female population in particular. In the span of only a single generation, primary and secondary education provided by the state of Israel sent illiteracy rates plummeting, from 95% in 1949 to 25% in 2014; those still illiterate are aged 55 and above (Ben-David, 1999, p.1; Interagency Task Force on Israeli Arab Issues Fact Sheet, 2014, p.1).

According to Ben-David (1999), between thirty and fifty percent of the students in Negev Bedouin elementary schools continue on to high school, a ratio similar to that found throughout the country's Arab sector. These students attend Bedouin high schools in the Negev and Arab high schools in the central and northern regions of the country (Ben-David, 1999). Nonetheless, matriculation exam levels in the Bedouin community are the lowest among all Arab-sector Israeli schools (28.2% in 2010, compared to 38.9% and 54.4% in the Arab and Jewish educational systems, respectively). The year 2011, however, saw an increase of 4.6% in the percentage of Bedouin students who passed their high school matriculation exams (Inter-Israeli Task Force on Israeli Arab Issues, 2014, p. 1).

And, critically, the outreach efforts of multiple programs of higher education targeting young women in this population have resulted in young Bedouin women enjoying a wide array of higher education choices (Al-Krenawi, 2013).

Nonetheless, there remains a large sector comprised of female Bedouin who 'fall through the cracks,' that is, girls who do not manage to acquire higher education, and, in fact, even drop out of secondary school. Abu-Rabia Queder (2007) sketches the creative manner in which this group manages to rebel against its parent system. The author approaches her topic of inquiry 'from the inside,' both as an Arab-Bedouin woman as well as by asking questions and listening to answers in such a way that her subjects were able to express themselves almost despite themselves. This was accomplished, according to the author, by being '...highly familiar with the specific cultural conditions of the group under study. (Abu-Rabia-Queder, 2007, p.186). As such, this ethnographic work models the best of the transcultural developments to date.

Noting that all Arab women in the Middle East are still strongly framed by patriarchal limitations, and that ignoring these might well endanger them socially and physically, Abu-Rabia Queder tackles what she terms the resistance strategies of 'invisible actions' (in contrast to 'visible actions' such as seeking support from family, using cultural/religious trappings as a cover for desired behavior, collaboration with political leadership, and female networking). Arrestingly, the author found that the Bedouin schoolgirl dropouts she studied *use thinking as a tool of resistance*. That is, these girls, who have been denied even completion of secondary education by often uneducated and unemployed fathers:

> ...struggle to maintain an autonomous spirit and consciousness. They express their resistance through their perceptions, through ways of thinking that differ from their parents' perceptions. This silent, implicit resistance is their own 'action.' (Abu-Rabia-Queder, 2007, p. 186).

In other words, as compared to the Bedouin schoolgirls who she studied, Abu-Rabia-Queder found that the Bedouin schoolgirl dropouts conform to particular traditional demands (e.g., dress codes), while defining that very conformance in ways that are at odds with the patriarchal context. This 'action,' as Abu-Rabia-Queder terms it, appears to be quite intersticial, falling between traditional notions of 'activity' and 'passivity' that are prescribed by Arab society at large for men and women, respectively. In the research set out below, we will gain a deeper sense of how this manifests itself in the Bedouin community of the Negev.

The Research: Symptom Reporting among Bedouin-Arab Women

As discussed above, it is culturally acceptable for Arab women in the Middle East to turn to a primary care clinic for help with somatic problems. In light of the global research on primary care use and the identification of emotional distress, we were interested in investigating the individual and familial distress of Bedouin-Arab women who approach primary care health clinics with bodily complaints. Further, bearing in mind the toll on women taken by divorce in the Arab world, we also decided to examine the characteristics of single, married and divorced women who report these symptoms.

In stage one of the research, the sample consisted of 217 Bedouin-Arab women from the town of Rahat, located in southern Israel. Convenience and snowball methods of recruiting were used. Forty-six percent of the women were single, 34% were married and 20% were separated, divorced or widowed. Their ages ranged from 16 to 85 (M=30, SD=13). Thirty-one percent had a primary school education, 13% had been graduated from middle school, 37% had received a high school diploma and 19% had studied in institutions of education. Eighty-one percent were unemployed, 6% were employed outside of their profession and 13% were employed in their profession.

In stage two of the research, 308 Bedouin-Arab women who had visited the health clinic in Rahat for medical care were recruited using convenience and snowball methods. Short interviews were conducted with the physicians who treated these women regarding their medical conditions. Thirty-two percent of the women were single, 36% married and 32% separated, divorced or widowed. Their ages ranged from 14 to 70 (M=30, SD=12), and their education ranged from 0 to 16 years of schooling (M=7, SD=5). Eighty-six percent were unemployed, 2% were employed outside of their profession and 12% were employed in their profession. Results were compared to those retrieved in the first stage.

In the third and final stage of the research, 30 women who complained of somatic symptoms were randomly selected from the previous sample, and interviewed at length. Ten of these women were single, 10 were married and 10 were separated, divorced or widowed. Their ages ranged from 16.5 to 62 (M=30, SD=11). Their education ranged from 0 to 15 years of schooling (M=11, SD=5). Fifty-two percent were unemployed, 19% were students (high school or university) and 29% were employed.

Data Collection

The questionnaires administered in the first two stages consisted of closed questions and standard research instruments. In the third stage, semi-structured, open-ended interviews were conducted. Bedouin-Arab female university students from the Negev conducted the interviews. The subjects were informed of the goals of the research and their agreement to participate in it was solicited. Each woman was interviewed individually; the answers were recorded by the interviewers on the questionnaires. In stage two of the research, interviews were conducted with the medical doctors in the primary care clinic. Subjects' social security numbers were used to identify the patients' medical file.

Research Instruments

The following instruments were used in the first two stages of research:

Demographic and behavioral variables

1. Participant's age, family status, age and number of children, type of marital structure (polygynous/monogynous), education, employment status, religious observance, housing status, economic status, husband's educational and employment status, age at marriage, marital relationship, duration of marriage, nutrition, number of friends to whom the woman turned in times of emotional need, feelings of isolation, number of visits to primary care clinic in the last week/ month, intensity of symptoms in the last month.
2. In Stage Two, physicians were asked: How often did the patient visit the clinic in the last month? What are her somatic complaints, and the intensity of her somatic complaints on a scale of 1-9? Did s/he think the patient was reacting in a somatic way to socio-emotional difficulties?

Emotional functioning

1. Self-esteem was measured with a standard questionnaire (Rosenberg, 1979). The Self-Esteem scale (SE) consists of 10 items and is easy

to complete. It has a high level of internal reliability (Gutman's measurement of reconstruction = 0.92) and a high test-retest reliability (r = 0.85). It also has high concurrent and construct validity. The internal reliability for the first stage of the current study was good (Cronbach's alpha= 0.79, N= 204). The internal reliability for the second stage was satisfactory (Cronbach's alpha= 0.76, N= 303).

2. Antonovsky's (1987) Sense of Coherence questionaire (SOC) was administered. This is a standard instrument consisting of 29 items; three theoretical dimensions are tested: comprehensibility, manageability, and meaningfulness. This questionnaire is used frequently in intercultural research. Here, we adapted the instrument to include only 13 items. The level of internal reliability of the SOC-13 found in 16 research studies in Israel and around the world is satisfactory (Cronbach's alpha= 0.74-0.91) (Antonovsky, 1993). Test-retest reliability exams show a reasonable level of stability (r=0.54), when the tests were administered two years apart. Further, the questionnaire was found to distinguish between healthy and neurotic populations (Antonovsky, 1987). The level of internal reliability for the first stage of the current study was satisfactory (Cronbach's alpha= 0.77, N= 193). The level of internal reliability for the second stage was also satisfactory (Cronbach's alpha= 0.78, N= 299).

3. Derogatis' (1977) SCL-90-R (Symptom Checklist) was also used. This questionnaire includes 90 items and 9 dimensions of psychological functioning: somatization, obsession-compulsion, interpersonal sensitivity, anxiety, hostility, paranoid ideation, panic (phobic anxiety), psychotism and depression. Internal reliability, measured in research among out-patients in US psychiatric clinics, was high (Cronbach's alpha= 0.78-0.90) and test-retest reliability was satisfactory (0.68-0.84) (Horowitz, Rosenberg, Baer, Ureno & Villasenor, 1988, cited in Derogatis, 1992). The questionnaire has a reasonable level of validity that was measured in comparison to the MMPI questionnaire. All the dimensions were highly correlated with parallel constructs in the MMPI, except for the obsession-compulsion dimension, that has no parallel construct on the MMPI scale. The reliability levels of the SCL-90-R in the first stage of the current study were as follows: Somatization – alpha= 0.86, N=201. Obsession-compulsion – alpha= 0.63, N=139. Interpersonal sensitivity – alpha= 0.80, N=199. Anxiety – alpha= 0.85, N=201. Hostility – alpha= 0.76, N=203. Paranoid ideation – alpha= 0.72, N=205. Panic (phobic anxiety) – alpha= 0.77,

N=203. Psychotism – alpha= 0.79, N=201. Depression – alpha= 0.86, N=204. All the items together (GSI) – alpha= 0.96, N=114. The reliability levels of the SCL-90-R in the second stage of the current study were as follows: Somatization – alpha= 0.86, N=292. Obsession-compulsion – alpha= 0.86, N=220. Interpersonal sensitivity – alpha= 0.79, N=301. Anxiety – alpha= 0.83, N=303. Hostility – alpha= 0.72, N=304. Paranoid ideation – alpha= 0.77, N=301. Panic (phobic anxiety) – alpha= 0.80, N=303. Psychotism – alpha= 0.80, N=302. Depression – alpha= 0.87, N=298. All the items together (GSI) – alpha= 0.98, N=195.

Family Functioning

1. The McMaster Family Assessment Device (FAD), developed by Epstein and colleagues (Epstein et al., 1983; Miller et al., 1985) was administered. This questionnaire includes 60 items pertaining to seven dimensions of family functioning: problem solving, communication, familial roles, emotional involvement, behavior control, emotional responses and general functioning. All sub-scales range from 1- 4, with higher scores indicating a lower level of family functioning. While cut-off points discriminating between 'clinical' and 'normal' families in American populations are available, none exist for Israeli families. The scale has a satisfactory level of reliability (Cronbach's alpha = 0.72-0.92), good test-retest reliability (r = 0.66) and a high level of validity, as indicated by comparing the scale's scores to other measures of the same matters (Epstein et al., 1983; Miller, Epstein, Bishop, & Keitner, 1985). In this study we only analyzed the sub-scale 'general functioning' that has 12 questions. Ridenour et al. (1999) reported that these 12 questions alone were sufficient to determine level of family functioning. The reliability level of this sub-scale, in the first stage of the current study, was high (Cronbach's alpha= 0.85, N= 189). The reliability level of this sub-scale, in the second stage of the current study, was quite low (Cronbach's alpha= 0.68, N= 284).

Overall Life Satisfaction

1. We administered Diener et al.'s (1985) Satisfaction with life (SWLS). Theis 5-item questionnaire has a high level of internal reliability

(Cronbach's alpha= 0.87) and a good level of stability, measured by test-retest (r= 0.82). The validity of the questionnaire, measured by comparison to existing questionnaire scores, was good (Diener et al., 1985). The level of internal reliability in the first stage of the current study was satisfactory (Cronbach's alpha= 0.79, N=199), and it was also satisfactiory in the second stage (Cronbach's alpha= 0.76, N= 301). These results are in line with the reliability levels recorded in the literature for this questionnaire.

2. Marital satisfaction
    a. Closed questions pertaining to the participant's relationship with her husband were asked, including number of times per day, week or month the woman and husband spent time together, financial support provided by the husband, relationship with the children and emotional support.
    b. The Enrich questionnaire was administered. This questionnaire, which measures marital satisfaction and the quality of adjustment to it, is divided into 8 parts, each containing 10 items. (Fournier, Olson & Druckman, 1983, cited in Lavee et al., 1987) found that it has a high level of reliability (Cronbach's alpha = 0.88-0.89). Other studies have reported a high degree of discriminating validity and concurrent validity. The questionnaire was translated into Hebrew and adapted by [first name] Lavee at Haifa University. It contains 95 statements used for clinical discrimination. Work with the instrument in Arab communities in Israel (Lev-Wiesel & Al-Krenawi, 1999) reported a satisfactory level of internal reliability (Cronbach's alpha = 0.89, N = 291). In the current study we used the short version of the Enrich questionnaire, created by Yoav Lavee, that includes only 10 items. The level of internal reliability of the short version in the first stage is very high (Cronbach's alpha = 0.92, N = 74), while the level of internal reliability of the short version in the second stage is high (Cronbach's alpha = 0.92, N = 96).

In the third stage of the research, we conducted semi-structured, open-ended interviews using the Qualitative Research Method. Interviewers introduced topics on family and marital life, relationship with husband and extended family, arranged marriage, women's rights, motherhood, personal problems and suffering. A thematic analysis was conducted according to the Tutty, Rothery & Grinnell (1996) guidelines of identifying meaning units and categories and classifying them according to themes.

According to Holosko (2001), the Qualitative Research Method entails a description of persons in their natural surroundings, wherein the researcher is an active agent. As such, s/he begins with a wide-angle view and does not broach particular lines of inquiry with the subjects. As the interview progresses, s/he forms opinions of the research via her/his reactions to the experiences of her/his subjects.

Results

First Sample

Socio-demographic characteristics of the three groups

Table 1 presents the socio-demographic characteristics of the subjects in the three research groups. The results show that the single women were the youngest of the three groups, while the women who were separated, divorced or widowed were the oldest ($P<.001$). The single women were the most educated (34% had had high-school educations, in comparison to 10% of the married women and 4% of the women who were separated, divorced or widowed), while the women who were separated, divorced or widows were the least educated (73% had only elementary school education, compared to 37% of the married women and 7% of the single women) ($P<.001$). The percentage of women who did not report religious observance was highest among the single women (43%, in comparison to 36% of the married women and 18% of the women who were separated, divorced or widowed). The percentage of women who reported religious observance is the highest among the women who were separated, divorced or widowed ($P<.05$).

Table 1
Socio-demographic characteristics of the three groups

Variable	Values	Entire sample N=217	Single N=99	Married N=74	Separated divorced or widowed N=44
Age***		M=31 SD=13	M=23 SD=6	M=33 SD=9	M=45 SD=15
Education ***	Elementary school	31%	7%	37%	73%
	Junior high school	13%	15%	13%	9%
	High school	37%	44%	40%	14%
	Higher education	19%	34%	10%	4%
Occupation	Unemployed	81%	72%	85%	93%
	Employed not in her profession	6%	9%	4%	5%
	Employed in her profession	13%	19%	11%	2%
Religious observance*	Practices	65%	57%	64%	82%
	Does not practice	35%	43%	36%	18%
Housing	Tent/hut	11%	12%	12%	9%
	Stone house	89%	88%	88%	91%
Place of residence	Out of the village	10%	11%	12%	2%
	In the village	90%	89%	88%	98%
Economic situation	Not good/not good at all	29%	29%	27%	29%
	Intermediate	35%	31%	43%	32%
	Good/very good	36%	40%	30%	39%
Primary aliments**	Sweets	5%	7%	1%	7%
	Dairy	19%	8%	24%	36%
	Meat	23%	19%	25%	29%
	Fruit and vegetables	15%	17%	17%	9%
	Bread, pasta, rise, potatoes	38%	49%	33%	19%

*P<0.05, **P<0.01, ***P<0.001

Behavioral-health characteristics of the three groups

Table 2 presents the behavioral-health characteristics of the subjects in the three research groups. Single women reported having the most close friends, while the women who were separated, divorced or widowed had the fewest (P<.05). The women who were separated, divorced or widowed expressed the strongest sense of loneliness (73% of them felt very much alone, in comparison to 15% of the married women and 25% of the single women). Loneliness was of least concern among the married women (57% of them never felt alone or only very seldom) (P<.001). In addition, married women had the strongest sense of having someone with whom to speak about their issues, while the women who were separated, divorced or widowed had the weakest sense (36% of them felt that they had no one with whome to talk about their problems, in comparison to 18% of the married women and 22% of the single women) (P<.05). Additional differences were found between the groups in the area of health. The married women complained of stomachaches (P<.05) and vomiting (P<.01) more frequently than the other two groups. In contrast, the separated, divorced or widowed participants complained of shortness of breath (P<.001), chest pressure (P<.01) and weakness (P<.01) more than the other two groups. This group also stands out with regard to other symptoms: its general symptom mean was the highest, although these differences were not significant. Furthermore, married women visited the clinic relatively frequently, but this difference was also not significant.

Table 2
Behavioral-health characteristics of the three groups

Variable	Values	Entire sample N=217	Single N=99	Married N=74	Separated, divorced or widowed N=44
Have 3 meals a day	Never/rarely	30%	28%	37%	23%
	Sometimes	31%	28%	28%	45%
	Often/always	39%	44%	35%	32%
No. of close friends*		M=2.4 SD=2.6	M=3 SD=3	M=2 SD=2.4	M=1.9 SD=1.9
Who she turns to in need	Husband	11%		31%	
	Relative	52%	50%	55%	55%
	Professional	4%	4%		11%
	Other	33%	46%	14%	34%

Sense of loneliness***	Never/a little Intermediate Often/very much	45% 24% 31%	51% 24% 25%	57% 28% 15%	14% 13% 73%
Sense of having someone to talk to about a problem*	Never/a little Intermediate Often/very much	48% 29% 23%	55% 23% 22%	49% 33% 18%	32% 32% 36%
No. of visits to the clinic in the last week		M=0.65 SD=1	M=0.65 SD=1.3	M=0.8 SD=1	M=0.45 SD=0.7
No. of visits to the clinic in the last month		M=1.2 SD=2.1	M=1.2 SD=2.5	M=1.6 SD=1.8	M=0.8 SD=1.5
No. of visits to a specialist in the last week		M=0.45 SD=1	M=0.5 SD=1.2	M=0.5 SD=0.95	M=0.3 SD=0.9
No. of visits to a specialist in the last month		M=0.9 SD=3	M=0.8 SD=3	M=1 SD=2	M=0.9 SD=3.2
Symptoms in the last month and severity					
Stomachache*		M=3.2 SD=2.4	M=3.1 SD=2.4	M=3.7 SD=2.6	M=2.5 SD=1.95
Nausea		M=3.3 SD=2.7	M=3.45 SD=2.7	M=3.4 SD=2.9	M=2.5 SD=2.9
Dizziness		M=3.7 SD=2.8	M=3.5 SD=2.8	M=3.6 SD=2.6	M=4.4 SD=3.1
Vomiting**		M=2.1 SD=2	M=1.8 SD=1.7	M=2.8 SD=2.5	M=1.7 SD=1.4
Over -Perspiration		M=2.45 SD=2.1	M=2.4 SD=1.9	M=2.4 SD=2.3	M=2.6 SD=2.4
Headaches		M=4.7 SD=2.8	M=4.6 SD=2.7	M=4.6 SD=2.85	M=5.2 SD=2.65
Shortness of breath***		M=3 SD=2.8	M=2.7 SD=2.6	M=2.5 SD=2.4	M=5.1 SD=3.3
Chest pressure**		M=3 SD=2.55	M=2.7 SD=2.3	M=2.6 SD=2.4	M=4.5 SD=2.9
Weakness**		M=4.25 SD=2.9	M=4.1 SD=2.9	M=3.8 SD=2.75	M=5.7 SD=2.8
General mean of the symptoms		M=3.33 SD=1.66	M=3.23 SD=1.73	M=3.32 SD=1.80	M=3.57 SD=1.19

*P<0.05, **P<0.01, ***P<0.001

1- weakest
9 - strongest

Demographic and behavioral characteristics of the married women

Table 3 presents the demographic and behavioral characteristics of the married participants. The results show that the average age of marriage is relatively young (19.7). Most of the women had an arranged marriage (65%). Further, most of the women and their husbands (74%) shared a blood relation. Forty-two percent of the participants were in polygamous marriages, and most of those were the second wife of their husband (55%). A large majority of participants in polygamous relationships (81%) reported conflict with the husband around the polygamy. Most women spent time together with their husband and children (88%), but only a minority spent time alone with their husband, without the children (42%).

Table 3
Demographic-behavioral characteristics of married women

Variable	Values	N=74
Is she pregnant	Yes No	28% 72%
Age at marriage		M=19.7 SD=3
No. of married years		M=13.5 SD=9.6
Husband's education	Elementary Junior high school High school Higher education	46% 15% 21% 18%
Husband's occupation	Unemployed Employed - not in his profession Employed - in his profession	27% 22% 51%
Type of marriage	Woman's choice Family's choice/ exchange marriage Other	42% 56% 2%
Relative of the husband	Not related Related	26% 74%
Polygamy	No Yes	58% 42%
No. of wife for this husband	1 2 3	32% 55% 13%

Relationship with husband's second/last wife	Not good at all/not good Average Good/very good	35% 39% 26%
Relationship with children of husband's second/last wife	Not good at all/not good Average Good/very good	13% 35% 52%
Fights with husband about second/last wife	Yes No	81% 19%
Does the husband stay the night at her house	Yes No	99% 1%
Does the husband discriminate among his wives	Not at all/no Intermediate Yes/very much	19% 32% 49%
No. of children		M=5.2 SD=3.6
No. of boys		M=2.8 SD=2.4
No. of girls		M=2.5 SD=2
Does the husband play with the children	No Yes	2% 98%
Do spouses go out with their children	No Yes	12% 88%
Do spouses go out alone	No Yes	58% 42%
Is the husband present at her house at night	No Yes	1% 99%

Emotional functioning, family functioning and overall life satisfaction of the three groups

Table 4 presents the emotional and family functioning and life satisfaction of the participants in the three research groups. As can be seen, in comparison to the single and married women, the women who were separated, divorced or widowed reported greater distress on several mental health dimensions: somatization (P<.001), paranoid ideation (P<.05), GSI (P<.05) and PSDI (P<.05). The mean of the family functioning scale for this sample (2.15) more closely resembles the clinical mean found in the American sample (2.26) than the non-clinical mean (1.96) found in the same sample (Epstein et al., 1983).

The correlation between marital satisfaction and education was found to be negative; that is, as educational levels rose, marital problems declined. However, that correlation was not significant.

Table 4
Emotional and family functioning and overall life satisfaction of the three groups

	Reliability	Entire sample N=217	Single N=99	Married N=74	Separated, divorced or widowed N=44	F values
Mental health[1]						
Somatization ***	0.86 N=201	M=1.42 SD=0.83	M=1.15 SD=0.8	M=1.48 SD=0.75	M=1.96 SD=0.75	F=16.58
Obsession-compulsion	0.63 N=139	M=1.75 SD=0.75	M=1.71 SD=0.78	M=1.67 SD=0.73	M=1.94 SD=0.65	F=1.97
Depression	0.86 N=204	M=1.73 SD=0.85	M=1.76 SD=0.93	M=1.59 SD=0.73	M=1.92 SD=0.81	F=2.19
Interpersonal sensitivity	0.80 N=199	M=1.77 SD=0.86	M=1.73 SD=0.90	M=1.81 SD=0.84	M=1.80 SD=0.80	F=0.19
Anxiety	0.85 N=201	M=1.54 SD=0.87	M=1.48 SD=0.94	M=1.49 SD=0.80	M=1.77 SD=0.79	F=1.87
Hostility	0.76 N=203	M=1.34 SD=0.97	M=1.31 SD=1.05	M=1.30 SD=0.83	M=1.50 SD=1.00	F=0.68
Phobic anxiety (panic)	0.77 N=203	M=1.46 SD=0.93	M=1.33 SD=0.89	M=1.44 SD=0.93	M=1.79 SD=0.97	F=3.75

Paranoid ideation*	0.72 N=205	M=1.83 SD=0.92	M=1.88 SD=0.98	M=1.69 SD=0.89	M=1.93 SD=0.83	F=1.27
Psychotism	0.79 N=201	M=1.39 SD=0.80	M=1.37 SD=0.88	M=1.27 SD=0.72	M=1.62 SD=0.72	F=2.59
GSI*	0.96 N=114	M=1.59 SD=0.70	M=1.52 SD=0.76	M=1.53 SD=0.65	M=1.84 SD=0.62	F=3.24
PST		M=59.64 SD=21.86	M=56.11 SD=21.24	M=61.22 SD=20.14	M=65.05 SD=24.94	F=2.83
PSDI*		M=2.36 SD=0.63	M=2.39 SD=0.64	M=2.2 SD=0.58	M=2.54 SD=0.66	F=4.09
Self-esteem[2]	0.79 N=204	M=2.98 SD=0.49	M=2.98 SD=0.53	M=2.99 SD=0.44	M=2.99 SD=0.45	F=0.002
Sense of coherence[3]	0.77 N=193	M=4.15 SD=1.00	M=4.10 SD=1.13	M=4.25 SD=0.88	M=4.10 SD=0.88	F=0.49
Family functioning[4]	0.85 N=189	M=2.15 SD=0.58	M=2.18 SD=0.59	M=2.17 SD=0.51	M=2.05 SD=0.68	F=0.76
Life satisfaction[5]	0.79 N=199	M=4.08 SD=1.48	M=4.08 SD=1.49	M=4.16 SD=1.45	M=3.94 SD=1.56	F=0.29
Marital satisfaction[6]	0.92 N=74			M=2.42 SD=0.96		

P<0.05, **P<0.01, ***P<0.001

1. The scale ranges from 0-4 with higher value indicating more mental health problems
2. The scale ranges from 1-4 with higher value indicating higher self-esteem
3. The scale ranges from 1-7 with higher value indicating a stronger sense of coherence
4. The scale ranges from 1-4 with higher value indicating more problems in family functioning
5. The scale ranges from 1-7 with higher value indicating more satisfaction with life
6. The scale ranges from 1-5 with higher value indicating less satisfaction with marriage

Second Sample

Socio-demographic characteristics of the three groups

Table 5 presents the socio-demographic characteristics of the participants in the three research groups. As can be seen, single women were the youngest of the three group, while the women who were separated, divorced or widowed were the oldest (P<.001). The single women were the most educated of those sampled, whereas the women who were separated, divorced or widowed were the least educated (P<.001). The percentage of religiously non-observant women is highest among the single women (42%, in comparison to 28% of the married women and 26% of the women who were separated, divorced or widowed). The percentage of religiously observant women was highest among the women who were separated, divorced or widowed (P<.05). As well, the financial situation of the women who were separated, divorced or widowed was the worst of all the groups: 53% of them described their financial situation as 'not good' or 'not good at all,' in comparison to 29% of the single women and 23% of the married women (P<.001).

Table 5
Socio-demographic characteristics of the three groups

Variable	Values	Entire sample N=308	Single N=99	Married N=110	Separated divorced or widowed N=99
Age***		M=30 SD=12	M=20.8 SD=5.1	M=28.2 SD=8.5	M=40.7 SD=11.3
Education ***		M=7.2 SD=5.1	M=10.7 SD=3.6	M=7.2 SD=4.9	M=4.1 SD=4.5
Occupation	Unemployed	86%	75%	88%	96%
	Employed-not in her profession	2%	6%	1%	
	Employed-in her profession	12%	19%	11%	4%
Religious observance*	Practices	68%	58%	72%	74%
	Does not practice	32%	42%	28%	26%
Housing	Tent/hut	9%	5%	12%	9%
	Stone house	91%	95%	88%	91%
Place of residence	Out of the village	8%	9%	8%	8%
	In the village	92%	91%	92%	92%
Economic situation ***	Not good/not good at all	34%	29%	23%	53%
	Intermediate	24%	26%	28%	17%
	Good/very good	42%	45%	49%	30%
Primary aliments**	Sweets	6%	12%	5%	1%
	Dairy	11%	17%	8%	9%
	Meat	18%	11%	18%	27%
	Fruit and vegetables	23%	28%	25%	16%
	Bread, pasta, rise, potatoes	41%	32%	45%	47%

*P<0.05, **P<0.01, ***P<0.001

Behavioral-health characteristics of the three groups

Table 6 presents the behavioral-health characteristics of the participants in the three research groups. We can see that the separated, divorced and widowed women expressed the strongest sense of loneliness (42% of them felt 'very much alone,' in comparison to 32% of the married women and 26% of the single women). Loneliness was found to be least burdensome among the married women (55% of them never felt lonely, or only infrequently) (P<.05). Separated, divorced and widowed women reported the strongest sense of not having someone with whom to discuss problems (30% of them felt they had no one to talk to about their problems, in comparison with 18% of the married women and 17% of the single women). These differences, however, were not significant.

Moreover, help-seeking patterns varied among groups: the single women sought support largely from their family members (92% in comparison to 35% of the married women and 34% of the women who were separated, divorced or widowed). The married women generally turned to their husbands (38%), while many of the women who were separated, divorced or widowed reported that they sought emotional assistance from someone 'other' than the individuals mentioned (42%) (P<.001).

Additional differences were found between the groups in the area of health behavior. Of all the groups, the married women reported the most difficulty with dizziness (P<.01). The separated, divorced or widowed participants complained more than the other groups of shortness of breath (P<.05), chest pressure (P<.05), weakness (P<.05), over-perspiration (P<.001) and headaches (P<.05). Further, the general mean of the symptoms for this group was the highest (P<.001). Women who were separated, divorced or widowed visited the clinic slightly more often than the other two groups, but the difference is not significant.

Nutrition constituted another point of variance: more single women never, or rarely, ate three meals per day, in comparison to the other two groups. In addition, more married women ate three meals per day, often or always, in comparison to the other two groups (P<.001).

Table 6
Behavioral-health characteristics of the three groups

Variable	Values	Entire sample N=308	Single N=99	Married N=110	Separated, divorced or widowed N=99
Have 3 meals a day**	Never/rarely Sometimes Often/always	32% 31% 37%	42% 34% 24%	27% 24% 49%	27% 36% 37%
No. of close friends		M=3.2 SD=3.3	M=3.3 SD=3.2	M=3.6 SD=4	M=2.7 SD=2.5
Who she turns to in need***	Husband Relative Professional Other	19% 44% 5% 32%	 62% 5% 33%	38% 35% 4% 23%	18% 34% 7% 41%
Sense of loneliness*	Never/a little Intermediate Often/very much	50% 17% 33%	53% 21% 26%	55% 13% 32%	40% 18% 42%
Sense of having someone to talk to about a problem	Never/a little Intermediate Often/very much	56% 22% 22%	62% 21% 17%	59% 23% 18%	47% 23% 30%
No. of visits to the clinic in the last week		M=1.5 SD=1.4	M=1.4 SD=1.3	M=1.5 SD=1.4	M=1.6 SD=1.5
No. of visits to the clinic in the last month		M=2.6 SD=3	M=2.2 SD=2.1	M=2.7 SD=3.3	M=2.8 SD=3.4
No. of visits to a specialist in the last week		M=0.3 SD=0.9	M=0.3 SD=1.0	M=0.3 SD=0.6	M=0.4 SD=0.9
No. of visits to a specialist in the last month		M=0.5 SD=1.2	M=0.5 SD=1.2	M=0.5 SD=1.3	M=0.5 SD=1.2
Symptoms in the last month and severity					
Stomachaches		M=4.4 SD=3.2	M=4.5 SD=3.2	M=4.5 SD=3.3	M=4 SD=3.1
Nausea		M=4.2 SD=3.1	M=3.7 SD=3	M=4.3 SD=3.3	M=4.4 SD=3
Dizziness**		M=4.9 SD=3.2	M=3.9 SD=3	M=5.4 SD=3	M=5.3 SD=3.3
Vomiting		M=3 SD=2.9	M=2.5 SD=2.5	M=3 SD=2.9	M=3.4 SD=3
Over – Perspiration ***		M=4.8 SD=3.3	M=3.8 SD=3	M=5 SD=3.4	M=5.7 SD=3.2

Table 6
Behavioral-health characteristics of the three groups (continued)

Headaches *		M=5.6 SD=3	M=5 SD=3.3	M=5.7 SD=3	M=6 SD=2.9
Shortness of breath*		M=3.5 SD=3	M=2.9 SD=2.7	M=3.4 SD=3.1	M=4 SD=3.2
Chest pressure*		M=3.7 SD=3	M=3.3 SD=2.9	M=3.5 SD=3	M=4.3 SD=3
Weakness*		M=3.9 SD=3.1	M=3.1 SD=2.8	M=4.1 SD=3.2	M=4.4 SD=3.2
General mean of the symptoms**		M=4.2 SD=2	M=3.7 SD=2	M=4.3 SD=2.1	M=4.7 SD=1.9

*P<0.05, **P<0.01, ***P<0.001

1- weakest

9- strongest

Demographic and behavioral characteristics of the married women

Table 7 presents the demographic and behavioral characteristics of the married paraticipants. As can be seen, the average age of marriage is relatively young (18.9). A majority of participants reported that they had had a say in choosing their spouses (61%); only a minority had participated in an exchange marriage or had married a person chosen by their family (38%). A blood relation existed between most of the women and their husbands (67%).

Thirty-six percent of the participants were in polygamous relationships, out of which 49% were the husband's first wife and 43% were his second wife. Most married women reported spending time outside of the house with their husband and children (65%), but only a handful reported time outside of the home spent exclusively with the husband (44%).

Table 7
Demographic-behavioral characteristics of the married women

Variable	Values	N=110
Patient pregnant	Yes No	22% 78%
Age at marriage		M=18.9 SD=3
No. of years married		M=10.3 SD=10.3
Husband's education		M=8.6 SD=4.9
Husband's occupation	Unemployed Employed - not in his profession Employed - in his profession	44% 24% 32%
Marital choice	Woman's choice Family's choice/ exchange marriage Other	61% 38% 1%
Relative of the husband	Not related Related	33% 67%
Polygamy	No Yes	64% 36%
No. of wife for this husband	1 2 3	49% 43% 8%

Relationship with husband's subsequent	Not good at all/not good Average Good/very good	17% 17% 66%
Relationship with children of husband's second/last wife	Not good at all/not good Average Good/very good	15% 9% 76%
Fights with husband about second/last wife	Yes No	36% 64%
Does the husband stay the night at her house	Yes No	92% 8%
Does the husband discriminate among his wives	Not at all/no Intermediate Yes/very much	35% 9% 56%
No. of children		M=3.5 SD=3
No. of boys		M=1.8 SD=1.9
No. of girls		M=1.8 SD=1.8
Does the husband play with the children	No Yes	5% 95%
Do spouses go out with their children	No Yes	35% 65%
Do spouses go out alone	No Yes	56% 44%
Is the husband present at her house at night	No Yes	3% 97%

Emotional and family functioning and overall life satisfaction of the three groups

Table 8 presents the emotional and family functioning and life satisfaction of the participants in the three research groups. While there are no significant differences between the groups on these scales, several trends can be noted. First, regarding mental health, on all scales except interpersonal sensitivity, the single participants scored lower than the other groups, pointing to fewer emotional problems. In comparison to the other groups, the separated, divorced or widowed participants reported higher rates of obsession-compulsion, interpersonal sensitivity, anxiety, phobic anxiety and psychotism. The married women reported the most somatization, depression and paranoid ideation. The separated, divorced or widowed women also reported the most problematic family functioning and the lowest levels of satisfaction with life. However, these differences were not statistically significant.

The mean of the family functioning scale for this sample (2.26) is identical to the clinical mean found in the American sample, and very different than the non-clinical mean (1.96) found in the same sample (Epstein et al., 1983).

Table 8

Emotional functioning, family functioning and overall life satisfaction of the three groups

	Reliability	Entire sample N=308	Single N=99	Married N=110	Separated, divorced or widowed N=110	F values
Mental health[1]						
Somatization	0.86 N=292	M=1.36 SD=0.92	M=1.2 SD=0.83	M=1.45 SD=0.97	M=1.41 SD=0.96	F=1.97
Obsession-compulsion	0.86 N=220	M=1.38 SD=0.95	M=1.32 SD=0.91	M=1.4 SD=0.97	M=1.43 SD=0.98	F=0.32
Depression	0.87 N=298	M=1.42 SD=0.94	M=1.34 SD=0.94	M=1.5 SD=0.94	M=1.4 SD=0.93	F=0.76
Interpersonal sensitivity	0.79 N=301	M=1.37 SD=0.88	M=1.35 SD=0.93	M=1.34 SD=0.88	M=1.4 SD=0.85	F=0.25
Anxiety	0.83 N=303	M=1.36 SD=0.92	M=1.29 SD=0.93	M=1.39 SD=0.92	M=1.41 SD=0.91	F=0.54
Hostility	0.72 N=304	M=1.14 SD=0.91	M=1.1 SD=0.96	M=1.18 SD=0.93	M=1.18 SD=0.86	F=0.38
Phobic anxiety (panic)	0.80 N=303	M=1.15 SD=0.98	M=1.1 SD=0.94	M=1.16 SD=0.98	M=1.19 SD=1.02	F=0.24

Table 8
Emotional functioning, family functioning and overall life satisfaction of the three groups (continued)

Paranoid ideation	0.77 N=301	M=1.32 SD=0.99	M=1.29 SD=0.95	M=1.36 SD=1.03	M=1.31 SD=0.99	F=0.14
Psychotism	0.80 N=302	M=1.02 SD=0.82	M=0.95 SD=0.75	M=1.03 SD=0.87	M=1.08 SD=0.83	F=0.68
GSI	0.98 N=195	M=1.3 SD=0.81	M=1.23 SD=0.80	M=1.34 SD=0.83	M=1.33 SD=0.8	F=0.51
PST		M=47.37 SD=22.39	M=46.2 SD=22.49	M=47.2 SD=21.7	M=48.72 SD=23.18	F=0.32
PSDI		M=2.34 SD=0.76	M=2.24 SD=0.79	M=2.42 SD=0.76	M=2.36 SD=0.74	F=1.39
Self-esteem[2]	0.76 N=303	M=2.16 SD=0.47	M=2.14 SD=0.45	M=2.17 SD=0.51	M=2.15 SD=0.46	F=0.14
Sense of coherence[3]	0.78 N=299	M=4.23 SD=0.95	M=4.15 SD=0.93	M=4.25 SD=0.96	M=4.27 SD=0.95	F=0.44
Family functioning[4]	0.68 N=284	M=2.26 SD=0.41	M=2.26 SD=0.42	M=2.23 SD=0.44	M=2.29 SD=0.36	F=0.41
Life satisfaction[5]	0.76 N=301	M=4.0 SD=1.6	M=3.97 SD=1.46	M=4.2 SD=1.68	M=3.96 SD=1.63	F=0.78
Marital satisfaction[6]	0.92 N=96			M=2.44 SD=1		

1. The scale ranges from 0-4, with higher values indicating more mental health problems
2. The scale ranges from 1-4 with higher values indicating higher self-esteem
3. The scale ranges from 1-7, with higher values indicating a stronger sense of coherence
4. The scale ranges from 1-4, with higher values indicating a lower level of family functioning
5. The scale ranges from 1-7, with higher values indicating more satisfaction with life
6. The scale ranges from 1-5 with higher value indicating less satisfaction with marriage

Physicians' reports

In Table 9 we presented the reports of the physicians who treated the participants at the primary care facility. As can be seen, the single women reported the greatest number of somatic symptoms, and the married women reported the fewest (P<.001). Importantly, according to the physicians' reports, the measure in which the patient responded somatically to emotional problems was highest for the separated, divorced and widowed women, and lowest for the married women (P<.001). Further, as illustrated in the table, the separated, divorced and widowed women went most frequently to the clinic – with a mean of 2.27 visits in the preceding month, in comparison to 1.88 for the single women and 1.9 of the married women. However, this difference was not significant.

Table 9
Treating physicians' report

Variable	Entire sample N=308	Single N=99	Married N=110	Separated, divorced or widowed N=110
Intensity of somatic complaints***	M=4.68 SD=2.3	M=5.92 SD=2.05	M=3.72 SD=2.09	M=4.54 SD=2.24
Measure of somatic reaction to emotional problems***	M=3.62 SD=2.37	M=3.70 SD=2.32	M=2.96 SD=2.15	M=4.29 SD=2.49
No. of visits to the clinic in the last month	M=2.01 SD=1.59	M=1.88 SD=1.34	M=1.9 SD=1.82	M=2.27 SD=1.54

Third sample

The single and the married women interviewed in this phase of the study were relatively young: among the single participants, the average age was 22.5, and among married participants it was 26.3. The third group, the divorced, separated or widowed women, were older: the age average of this group was 40.

Among the married women, one was in a polygamous marriage and four of the single women were from polygamous families. The rate of polygamy among the divorced, separated or widowed women could not be determined.

Single women

Six of the participants complained of bodily symptoms: five participants reported headaches, and one complained of overall physical weakness. The attribution of these problems varied: two women ascribed them to the 'evil eye,' one to her educational workload, three to household work, and one to social problems.

Most of the women (8 of 10) expressed positivity toward intra-tribal marriage.

Two women said they were not currently considering marriage, one stated that she was interested in being married, and one was engaged.

Six women reported good relationships in their families. One participant stated that although she had problems with her father, she was close with her other family members.

Five women expressed the opinion that the status of women in the Arab-Bedouin society is in need of reform. Three participants spoke of discomfort with women's status in Bedouin society in general, but not in their families. One interviewee stated that she was satisfied with women's status in Bedouin society.

Divorced, separated or widowed women

Most of the women (8 of 10) complained of symptoms of some sort: six women mentioned pain of some kind (headache in two cases), and four women spoke of exhaustion or an overall sense of weakness. Three women reported strong anxiety.

Five women specified distress around their poor economic situation.

In addition, three women stated distress around past or present living conditions.

Half the women said they had never completed their obligatory studies (9 years of schooling). Two interviewees were analphabetic.

Three women stated an interest in bearing more children, while two interviewees stated that theßy did not wish to bear more children.

Married women

Interviewees were permitted to raise topics of their choice. Fifty percent of the participants began the discussion with the subject of their children, two with their medical condition, two with their marriage and one with her economic situation. Sixty percent of the women eventually brought up financial difficulties.

Sixty percent of the women complained of body pain. The most frequent complaints were leg and head pain; these were typically described in combination with pain in other areas of the body. Pregnancy and childbirth was offered as the source of somatic pain by fifty percent of the women; twenty percent attributed the pain to work, one to her financial situation, and one declined to specify.

Qualitative Findings

The qualitative findings were based on two samples and a total of more than 500 women. The two samples, similar in many respects, were marked nonetheless by some notable differences.

The separated, divorced or widowed group constituted the least educated, most religious and poorest of all the groups. They presented as having few friends; hence, few with whom to discuss their physical and emotional problems. Importantly, these women also scored the highest (indicating more distress) on most dimensions of the mental health scale.

In addition, this third group reported many more somatic symptoms compared to the married and single women, and the severity of these symptoms was high, as compared to the other two groups. Moreover, the physicians' reports reveal that these participants manifested the highest degree of somatic reaction to emotional problems.

More than a third of the married women in both samples were in polygamous marriages. Surprisingly, in the second sample, the majority of the women in polygamous marriages reported marital satisfaction, while in the first sample the reports of these women are far less positive. This finding may be attributed to the fact that in the second sample the majority of women in polygamous marriages were the second wife of the husband, while the majority of the women in polygamous marriages in the first sample were their husband's first wife. The literature indicates that first and subsequent wives in polygamous marriages experience polygamy differently. Among Bedouin-Arabs, first marriages are commonly arranged by parents/elders consanguineous or by exchange (where two men are married to each other's sister) (Chaleby, 1985; El-Islam, 1989; Al-Krenawi, 2014). Subsequent marriages may be more choice-related. Hence, despite Islamic dictates, subsequent wives may enjoy a favored status with respect to economic resources and spousal regard (Al-Krenawi, 2013).

Quantitative Findings

The interviews conducted with three groups of Bedouin-Arab women who sought help at the Rahat primary care center enabled us to deepen our understanding of the somatic symptom reporting of the interviewees.

Married women spoke first of their children. This is consonant with the Arab focus on female fertility. An interesting sense of contradiction quickly arose in the interviews: these same women traced back a great deal of their physical pain to pregnancy and childbirth. The somatic emphasis of the mothers' complaints, then, deserves careful examination. Enculturated to dedicate their lives to their husband and children, these women are barred by cultural consensus to discuss domestic overload. They are permitted, however, to bring up bodily distress – and when they do, they tend to relate it to the travails of childbearing.

Financial distress was a universal complaint among the participants. However, this topic was especially salient among the married and the divorced, separated or widowed.

Typically, single women reported that they enjoyed good relations with their family members, and especially with their parents. Again, this report should be culturally contextualized. As noted earlier in this volume, as well as in subsequent chapters, the overarching Arab mores of family honor, and honor toward elders in particular, may well be at play here. Women whose father was engaged in polygamous relations reported relatively poor familial relationships. This finding is in line with a great deal of literature on polygamy (Al-Krenawi, 2013).

Reflecting the process of acculturation in which the Bedouin-Arab society is engaged, half of the single female interviewees stated that they were dissatisfied with the status of women in their community. Tellingly, however, none of the women volunteered the notion that changes needed to take place within their own homes.

The divorced, separated and widowed study participants highlighted their educational as well as educational straits: fifty percent disclosed that they had never completed their basic obligatory studies. Interestingly, many among this group refrained from revealing during the interview that they were divorced or separated, although they had reported their marital status while completing the questionnaire in the Rahat primary care center. The socially repugnant status of divorce, discussed at length later in this volume, may have made it difficult to broach this issue with a stranger.

Somatic complaints varied across groups in two dimensions: quality and type. As to the former, duration of distress was a distinguishing factor between complaints; as to the latter, the physical location of the distress served to demarcate the groups.

Single and married women reported specific, oftentimes temporary symptoms, with headache ranking first among single women and leg pain taking first place in the married group. The divorced, separated and widowed women, however, complained of generalized somatic issues such as exhaustion and enervation, and reported anxiety as well. Further, and in contrast with sporatic nature of pain described by the first two groups of interviewees, women in this third group described their symptoms as chronic.

In chapter eight, we will discuss the clinical implications of these findings, and present the comprehensive treatment model for Arab women in the Middle East that was constructed on its basis.

Chapter 9
Discussion and Clinical Implications: Toward a Transcultural Treatment Synthesis: Wrap-Around Resilience

Overview

In the previous chapter, we took up the question of how the idiom of distress of possession, prevalent among many traditional societies, manifests itself as 'al-junun' in the Arab region. In the present chapter, we will advance a step further and consider how Arab/Islamic conceptions of mental health and illness can be carefully leveraged for therapeutic gain among Arab women in the Middle East. Directive, goal-oriented, short-term modalities have been suggested as most appropriate for this population (Dwairy, 1998). Metaphor therapies, mindfulness treatments and family interventions, all of which may be described in the above terms, form the tripartite crux of this work. These techniques, used in the service of true cultural competency, may be fashioned to take into account the enculturation of the Arab female client. In this investigation, we will be moving a notch beyond what scholars have construed as recognizing 'culture only at the margins, in the encounter with those we view as 'different' or 'other" (Gone and Kirmayer, 2010, p. 90). Rather, we will be meeting the Arab client where she truly is.

Toward a transcultural treatment synthesis: Wrap-Around Resilience

In chapter seven, we described at length our research among Bedouin-Arab women in the Negev. While this is a specific sub-population in the Middle East, many of the elements that should be taken into account when formulating a treatment approach for the larger population of Arab women in the region emerge directly from that work. These points include highly sensitive primary care, which, when appropriate, would segue into culturally competent (and possibly traditional) psychological treatment, targeted attention to somatic symptom reporting and somatization issues, and planned, preemptive outreach toward Arab women who are experiencing marital distress or divorce.

These three crucial components of care for Arab women in the Middle East may form the fulcrum of an intervention policy that aims to meet the mental health needs of Arab women. In recognition of the comprehensive nature of the program (essentially, a pinpointed bio-psycho-social approach), we propose to term this policy 'Wrap-Around Resilience.' With this designation, we follow the work of scholars in the growing field of resilience research (Werner and Smith, 2005; Luthar, 2003).

Resilience has been defined as, '*the dynamic process encompassing positive adaptation within the context of significant adversity*' (Luthar, Cicchetti, and Becker, 2000, p. 543, emphasis in original, cited in Ungar, 2011, p. 1). Recently, scholars have begun to widen the lens of resilience research and take up the notion of the 'social ecological understanding of positive development' (Ungar, 2011, p.2). For instance:

> Because resilience is related to the presence of social risk factors, there is a need for an ecological interpretation of the construct that acknowledges the importance of people's interactions with their environments...This understanding of resilience extends the discourse concerning positive human development under adversity suggesting that social ecological factors such as family, school, neighborhood, community services and cultural practices are as influential as psychological aspects of development when individuals are under stress (Ungar, 2013, p.1).

The 'Wrap-Around Resilience' policy for women in the Arab region puts forward a strategic blend of the 'ecological factors' of the bio-medical primary care system, native healing practices, clinical work informed by somatic and metaphoric configurations of the self, and a rich program of outreach for both divorced Arab women and those in marital distress. Arab women in the Arab region live sociocentric lives; resilience research, and especially the 'nascent construct' of the social ecology of resilience (Ungar, 2011) has taught us the value of strengthening the individual from the outside in.

First component: Primary care and traditional treatments

Wrap-Around Resilience must be informed by what we know about the choices and beliefs prevalent in this region. Thus, proper primary care intervention constitutes a crucial, first-line approach to care for Arab women in the Middle East. For instance, it has been suggested that the biomedical system could provide pivotal identification of, and assistance to, victims of intimate partner violence (Boy & Kulczycki, 2008). In light of the rate of extended family violence in the region (Morse, et al., 2012), primary-care intervention could be critical in this realm as well. In like manner, physicians working in Arab-region primary care facilities might sharpen their awareness of the inclination toward the somatic expression of distress found among Arab women, and divorced Arab women in particular. The interdisciplinary aspect of primary care should not end, however, with a physician's referral to a social worker. Kirmayer (2003) has reminded us that, 'Intercultural work raises a series of dilemmas for the clinical encounter' (p. 249). As demonstrated in a growing body of research (Kirmayer, 2003; Al-Krenawi, 1998b, 2001, 2014), reasonable resolutions of these dilemmas, as well as the general efficacy of treatment in the Middle East hinges on the ability of the biomedical team to make flexible use of a variety of healers and techniques, including those located in the traditional sphere. This notion has reached the forefront of international healthcare strategy, as noted at a recent international conference on traditional medicine for South-East Asian countries, where WHO Director-General Dr. Margaret Chan stated that:

> ...traditional medicines, of proven quality, safety, and efficacy, contribute to the goal of ensuring that all people have access to care. For many millions of people, herbal medicines, traditional treatments, and traditional practitioners are the main source of health care, and sometimes the only source of care. This is care that is close to homes, accessible and affordable. It is also culturally acceptable and trusted by large numbers of people. The affordability of most traditional medicines makes them all the more attractive at a time of soaring health-care costs and nearly universal austerity. Traditional medicine also stands out as a way of coping with the relentless rise of chronic non-communicable diseases (Margaret Chan, WHO, 2013).

The above-noted passage clarifies beyond question that traditional approaches to healthcare are being taken with utmost seriousness by the leaders of the international medical community. Our proposed program of 'Wrap-Around Resilience' shows a great deal of congruence with this notion, and incorporates within it a call for complementary utilization of traditional mental health practices. Practically, this would mean having on staff (or on call) individuals who are familiar with the cultural and religious canons of Arab communities (Al-Krenawi, 2013), as well as individuals able to work hand-in-hand with traditional healers to effect a positive treatment outcome for Arab women (Al-Krenawi, 1998b, 2001, 2014). Especially in cases that involve multiple families and high stakes such as violence and divorce, community cultural mediators (*wasits*) may be used to bridge gaps between the biomedical system and the Arab home environment (Al-Krenawi & Graham, 2001). In all cases, clinicians with deep awareness of important cultural codes and belief systems in the Arab world would work to assist the other biomedical practitioners in intervening effectively with their female Arab patients.

Second component: Managing somatic symptom reporting

The somatic symptom reporting and somatization data that emerged from the research presented in chapter seven accords with the transcultural data we have on somatization and primary care treatment. The participants in the study, permitted by their cultural canon to seek medical help from the primary care physician, did just that – with a concomitant concentration on bodily complaints. Their language, however, betrayed a different sense, one of overburden and, in the case of divorced participants, loneliness. These feelings were not revealed in the primary care clinical interviews; rather, they remained under wraps until identified by both the qualitative and quantitative portions of the research. The behavior of the Arab-Bedouin subjects, however, was far from unusual in the MENA region. In an earlier chapter we mentioned Becker's (2004) finding that while Saudi primary care physicians are clearly aware of psychiatric disorders, they have a great deal of difficulty diagnosing somatization and depression. Importantly, the researcher noted that this situation may be explained, at least partially, by the fact that 'patients may express psychosocial problems in somatic terms both to themselves and to their doctor, making it difficult to detect psychiatric morbidity (Becker, 2004, p. 962). One final point of interest here is the apparent ubiquity of the behavior: the participants in Beck's above-mentioned work lived in an urban setting, namely, Riyadh, the capital city of Saudi Arabia. This finding supports the notion that we are not discussing here a strictly rural phenomenon.

One has the sense that female patients in the Arab region tend to speak in a kind of somatic code. Let us recall chapter five, where we read of the multiple and telling metaphors with which the participants expressed themselves. Too, consider Hinton and Lewis-Fernández (2010):

> Idioms matter…if a clinician does not recognize complaints as culture-specific idioms (i.e., as opening up a complex network of meanings…he or she may not attain a level of understanding of the patient's lifeworld [sic] critical to valid diagnostic practice and consensual treatment negotiation (p. 3).

The somatic codes and metaphors of Arab women are a sort of idiom, and, as these researchers note, even the most basic level of treatment agreement is contingent upon a clinician's awareness of the true import of a patient's 'complaints.' Without that knowledge, the patient and the clinician are speaking, literally, different languages.

As such, the second element in a comprehensive care program for Arab women in the Middle East might encompass training for bio-medical practitioners in 'decoding' the language of Arab women in distress. Idiom of distress decoding for women with somatic problems was the subject of a recent paper by de Jong and Reis (2010). The authors report on what they term a 'West-African postwar idiom of distress,' Kiyang-yang (p. 31). Discussing the metaphorical aspect of idioms of distress, the authors note:

> …an individual expression of distress can only develop into a legitimate idiom of distress if its language can be understood and appropriated by others… we argue that for this to happen, there has be some resonance at the level of symbolic language…as well as at the level of what it aims to communicate (e.g., the psychosocial suffering such as despair…). It is the *metaphorical* dimension of an idiom of distress that allows for resonance on different levels of experience…in the case of Kiyang-yang, the idiom allowed for a simultaneous embodied language for individual suffering…and the suffering of groups of marginalized women… (de Jong & Reis, 2010, p. 319).

While Kiyang-yang is related to a healing cult for infertile young women in southern Guinea Bissau (de Jong & Reis, 2010), it shares features with the somatic idiom of distress expressed by women in the Arab region. This 'embodied language,' as the authors put it, functions both for individual female patients as well as for groups of suffering women in the Middle East. In fact, the core somatic complaint (childbearing difficulties) and the core message (despair) are twin topoi for women in the Arab region.

To further broaden the perspective on some of the issues revealed in the study on somatic symptom reporting among Bedouin-Arab women, we present below two case examples. One of the case studies treats a Bedouin-Arab woman, while the other describes the somatic reporting of a Havic Brahmin woman. While they investigated samples in geographically divergent populations, both studies elucidate somatic symptom reporting as an idiom of distress among women at the culturally vulnerable moment of marital crisis.

Case Examples

Mass & Al-Krenawi's (1994) study on clinical relationships in Negev Bedouin-Arab society sheds light on the complexity of the somatization conundrum in this population. The authors note that as a male psychotherapist working in a primary health care clinic in southern Israel, Al-Krenawi had essentially broken the Bedouin social canon:

> ...the women were permitted to visit the clinic on the understanding that they went for medical treatment of physical symptoms. The permission did not encompass treatment based on close emotional ties between client and therapist...the professional relationship that had evolved was...taboo (Mass & Al-Krenawi, 1994, p. 262).

We note the clear and highly restrictive communal bounds of female Bedouin participation in the available biomedical system (i.e., somatic problems only) and concentrate on the somatic presentation of this case, as well as where it led. Al-Krenawi's patient, a divorced female, age 30, had come to the medical center with complaints of near-paralysis in her legs. No physical pathology could be determined. As the clinical intake progressed, the patient disclosed that at age 15 she had been 'given' to a man of sixty, who met her in a tent and raped her. The patient's parents were reported to have threatened the patient if she left her husband, which she did one year later, in the face of familial fury. When the patient's mother died some years later and the father remarried, the patient received and refused some proposals of marriage from male tribe members. The patient at this point began to experience leg pain. The authors suggest that the patient's 'paralysis... legitimated her dependent and debilitated status and her unsuitability for marriage' (Mass & Al-Krenawi, 1994, p. 361).

In this case study, we can recognize several elements that were raised in the larger study that forms the core of chapter seven, as well as some that have been highlighted throughout the book. The patient, a Bedouin-Arab female, was in her mid-teens when she was forced by her family to 'marry' a fellow tribe-member quadruple her age. Far from having consented to the union, the patient describes having been raped rather than wed. In light of the parental and communal pressure applied, the patient acquiesced to the relationship for one year, after which she divorced and, as was culturally expected, returned to her family of origin. Given what we now know about the depth of the 'honor' code among Arab societies, it is reasonable to speculate that the degree of familial recrimination with which this return was met reflected the perceived abrogation of 'honor' that now sullied the patient, as well as her family. The patient, now divorced, presented at the local medical clinic with the single type of distress that was culturally permitted to her: bodily ills.

Nichter (1981) offers an Indian case study that reveals more variations of the relationship between somatic symptomology and marital status issues. The context was one in which a Brahmin female, somewhat past culturally optimal marital age, became possessed after 'her initial somatic expression of distress, [which] focused attention upon her in a culturally legitimate manner' (p. 395) failed to achieve the hoped-for results: familial attention to her singlehood status. While in this instance, in contrast to the above-mentioned one, the patient actively (albeit unconsciously) sought the intervention of her family in matchmaking (by experiencing menstrual difficulties that were understood by the author to be meant to focus 'attention onto the girl's state of sexuality and vulnerability' (p. 395), the sense of the two cases is the same: female vulnerability and its associated distress around issues of marital status presenting itself in somatic complaints.

The proposed program goal of deciphering the somatic idioms of distress employed by Arab women in the Middle East must take into account that these idioms are multi-determined. For instance, as we have seen, in this region perceived female infertility, family violence, polygyny and divorce have been found to be highly interrelated (Morse et al., 2012). El-Saadani (2003) too found this among a wide range of women in Arab societies:

> Infertility in most of the Arab societies is considered a legitimate reason for divorce, especially if it is the wife who is infertile. Interestingly [sic] to notice that women themselves believe in it and even they are injustice toward themselves. A significant portion of the Egyptian women, as an illustration, (about one third) agrees that the husband has good [sic] reason to seek divorce if his wife was unable to have children and denies in [sic] the same time such right for the wife in case that her husband is responsible for childlessness. In contrast a much lower percent, 6.4%,

> agrees that the wife has good [sic] reason to seek divorce if the husband was unable to have children and denies such right for the husband in case that his wife is responsible for childlessness (El-Saadani, 2003, p. 14).

Thus, the somatic complaints made by women who experience these phenomena should be understood as potentially reflective of a wide range of psychosocial and physical ills. On a concrete level, Morse et al. (2012) suggests that when treating Arab individuals from the Middle East who are either infertile or who have no male offspring, private sessions should be held with each family member (including extended family) to determine how he or she is managing his or her feelings around those issues.

Third component: Outreach to divorced Arab women

The third component of a well-planned mental health care program for women in the Middle East would target a highly marginalized population in this region: divorced women. The research presented in chapter seven made quite evident the impact of divorce on the somatic complaints of the study participants. This dovetails with the other (albeit limited) research on divorce in this region. Some work has noted the intersectionality of infertility and divorce: 'Inability to bear children is a strong threat to marital stability' (El-Saadani, 2006, p. 23). Divorced Bedouin-Arab women are expected to return to their family of origin; that is, to their parents or, if they are no longer alive, to a close male family member. Hence, a woman's divorce becomes a full-family affair, likely to increase tension between the woman and her family of origin. Societal constructions of divorce further increase the complexity: a woman is typically assigned the blame for a 'failure' to keep her marriage intact (Brhoom, 1987). The heightened vulnerability of divorced Arab women, too, is addressed in the literature:

> Divorced women become [sic] vulnerable group of people who lacks support; emotionally, socially, and financially and suffers loss of their freedom and dignity (they [sic] subject to the authority of their fathers, mothers, and brothers) (El-Saadani, 2006, p. 1).

This loss of freedom endured by divorced women in the Arab region might be understood as a kind of double circumscription. In other words, the regulation of female sexuality, in normal circumstances a high priority in the Moslem Arab world, takes on even greater proportions in the case of divorced women, who may be perceived as a threat to the integrity of other families. As such, their freedom of movement outside of the home may be further limited (Al-Krenawi, 2014). El-Saadani's (2006) quote from the autobiography of a 'distinguished Moroccan writer' grants literary evidence of this notion:

> It was said – according to what has been kept in the memory of our friend, during his early childhood, ...It is in that time, around dawn time, when women return carrying water from water shields upper the hill and men go out washing for praying, one day, by chance or by prior arrangement that it happened quickly and secretly at one corner of the street, what could always happens between a man and a woman of prohibited sexual affairs...The truth is, this type or another of sexual affaires ... occurs very rarely, it is almost confined among some divorced men and women', (El-Gabry, M. Abed, 1997, pp.28-29, in Arabic, cited in El-Saadani, 2006, p. 1).

In El-Saadani's view, this quote well conveys the societal sense of stigma carried by divorced Arab individuals in general, and divorced Arab women in particular. Cohen and Savaya (1997), too, documented this sexual stigma in their pioneering work on the divorced woman in Moslem Arab society. The divorced female subjects in their study clarified that:

> ...their sexuality is called into question. Arab men apparently consider them fair game. Moreover, men are out to test them: 'People are like wolves, all the men make passes at me; they want to sleep with me. Even my own uncle sent some men to makes passes at me in order to test me' (Cohen & Savaya, 1997, p. 8).

It is worthy of note that the women in Cohen and Savaya's study were quite urbanized, residing as they did in a mixed Arab-Jewish neighborhood bordering Tel Aviv, Israel. Thus, while these subjects articulated views similar to those expressed by divorced Arab women in more rural and remote areas of the Arab region, they themselves were far from being geographically or culturally isolated.

Along these lines, El-Saadani's work on divorce trends in the Arab world also helps to broaden the aperture. Her research reflects an extraordinarily wide and substantive research base, based as it is on several decades of United Nations Demographic Yearbooks, as well as on the most recent national demographic surveys undertaken in all the countries of the Middle

East. This professor of demographics and biostatistics at Cairo University contends that for Arab women in the Arab region, professional success in no way makes up for failure in the marital arena. And, the bounds of this failure are quite broad: they include the notion that a woman is better off being married to *anyone at all* than to be living as a single woman. Offering an Arab proverb that strongly echoes the one with which we opened chapter three, El-Saadani (2006) tells us:

> The shadow of a wall is no better than the shadow of a man (El-Saadani, 2006, p. 1).

In the previously cited Arab proverb making a reference to a wall, the wall was a metaphor for sought-after but unfound safety. Here, according to El-Saadani:

> Such [sic] sentence teaches us that a woman would accept marrying to any one [sic] even if his sole role is not better than providing her a shadow (El-Saadani, 2006, p. 1).

The author punctuates her point with a pertinent line about polygamy:

> This concept is additionally reflected in the willingness of women (especially the divorced and celibate ladies) to be [sic] second wife in polygamy [sic] marriages (2006, p. 1).

In 1997, Cohen and Savaya reported that, 'divorced women say they are treated as pariahs and considered permanently deficient...They are referred to as 'broken glass,' from the Arab saying, 'glass once broken can never again be made whole' (p. 8). The current work of researchers such as El-Saadani (2006) informs us that the societal perception of the divorced Arab woman in the Arab region remains extremely degraded.

'Wrap-Around Resilience,' then, would serve to promote three crucial agendas for the mental health of Arab/Muslim women in the Arab region. First, and in keeping with the cultural canon of Arab societies, primary care would function as the gateway to a range of biomedical and traditional practitioners who would work in synergy to develop and carry out treatment plans for Arab women in the MENA region. This planning would take into careful account the interpersonal connectivity of such patients, on the micro (family), mezzo (extended family) and macro (tribe/community) levels. Second, the somatic symptom reporting and somatising behaviour of these populations would be considered a 'code' for communication of important bio-psycho-social distress, and the clinician, be she biomedical or traditional, would make a concerted effort to understand how the patient was using language, often metaphorical, to express this pain. This 'decoding' may well involve consultation with traditional practitioners. Finally, as we have seen, divorced Arab women in the Arab world contend with a range of physical, financial and attitudinal challenges. Our program would provide targeted outreach to this sector, which could also begin in the major setting for treatment in Arab region, as across the globe: primary care. As demonstrated above, each of the three points in our proposed tripartite program is in line with the strategies of current thought leaders in worldwide mental health. It is fitting, then, that at this juncture we turn to our concluding chapter, which limns some of the broader notions of theorists working in the fields of mental health and women's rights.

> 'Genetics, biochemistry, physiology, psychology, sociology, and anthropology are names for areas of human knowledge and inquiry. They are not, however, names for mutually exclusive events in nature...they are all relevant to the events we call psychiatric disorder.' Alexander Leighton, *My Name is Legion: The Stirling County Study*

Conclusion

The First Heave

Ezra Pound said in reference to Robert Frost, 'To break the pentameter, that was the first heave' (Columbia World of Quotations). In 1959, Alexander Leighton published the first volume of his path-blazing, three-volume work, *The Stirling County Study*. In making this first heave, Leighton and his colleagues midwifed the birth of cultural psychiatry. In time, and through the ministrations of the likes of Kleinman, Yap, Beiser, Kirmayer and others, cultural psychiatry was to become transcultural psychiatry ('old,' 'new' and 'beyond'; Kleinman, 1982; Kirmayer, 2006), then cultural psychiatry again, now imbued with a transnational consciousness, 'firmly committed to the presence of culture and context in every aspect of experience' (Kirmayer, 2014).

This volume represents an attempt to put these ideals into practice, in the specific case of Arab/Islamic women's mental health in the Middle East. We have aimed to take broad cognizance of the manifold interactions between culture and the well-being of women in this region. In other words, we have tried hard to consider the 'co-constitution of mind and culture' (Gone and Kirmayer, 2010, p. 79). To recall, Abu-Rabia Queder presented a striking instance of this 'co-constitution' in her ethnography of non-privileged Bedouin schoolgirls. She sought

> to show that women from the margins – that is, those who are not major actors in the public sphere and are essentially invisible – also have an individual face and, more importantly, have their own way of seeing their lives this both similar to and different from the educated girls (Abu-Rabia Queder, 2007, p. 162).

Thus, the author offered insight into 'ways of struggling that are invisible –those that fall in the arenas of language and consciousness rather than action' (p. 168). This type of response resonates radically with our work with women in the Bedouin-Arab community, as with that of Abu-Lughod. There, too, language became the conduit for the otherwise culturally verboten.

As well, we have explored the ways in which women's distress in the Arab world both parallels the distress of women across societies, as well as takes its own form, hewn by the particularities of Islamic/Arabic histories. Concretely, we have seen how constructions of honor in patriarchal societies have carved their initials on the bodies of Arab women, using the tools of forced and child marriage, of 'honor' killings, and, most literally, of the genital mutilation that ravages the Arabian Peninsula, Africa and southern Asia. And we have glimpsed a specific way in which the women of the Arab region have responded to these aspects of their culture: they have sung of their distress, clothing the call in the language of the body, which is anything but estranged from that pain. As it turns out, this 'somatic idiom of distress' perfectly suits the message. In this context of culture and personality, the psyche and the soma are of a piece.

Our research among Bedouin Arab women supports Kirmayer's (2008) view of the uses of metaphor and lyricism in the project of the expression of emotional anguish:

> It may be that the nonnarrative organization and intensity of metaphor and imagery of lyric poetry provides a better vehicle for communicating the texture of illness experience (Kirmayer, 2008, p. 464).

In fact, when our participants spoke their proverbs, or offered their somatic metaphors, they communicated their distress with extraordinary tonality.

Leila Ahmed, too, writes of language in the Arab region and beyond. In a paper on the recent educational development in the UAE and the concurrent abrogation of the local Bedouin culture, the Islamic scholar introduces the words of Kenyan writer Ngugi wa Thiong'o:

> Our appreciation of the suggestive magical power of language was reinforced by the games we played with words through...*proverbs*...(Ahmed, 2000, p. 87, italics added).

Thiong'o's mother tongue was:

> alive with 'the inflection of the voices of the people ... whose words had a 'suggestive power well beyond the immediate and lexical meaning' (Ahmed, 2000, p. 87).

In her article, Ahmed juxtaposes what she calls the 'Arab culture of literacy'; that is, the male-centered, medieval-based fundamentalist-driven textual history of things Islamic over what she maintains is a female-constructed, orally transmitted Islam of centeredness, flow and non-aggression. While doing so, she likens Thiong'o's account of his mother tongue to that of her own, that is, the vernacular Arabic (and Islam) that she absorbed from the matriarchs of her Egyptian family. Once again, we hear of proverbs, of the poetics of language, and especially, of the language of the mothers.

Going further into aurality, meaning and the body, Ahmed asserts:

> One might even argue that the oral tradition is intrinsic to Islam itself...The Quran was originally recited to the community by the Prophet Muhammad... Moreover, a bias in favor of the heard word, the word given life by the human voice, the human breath (*nafas*), is there, one might say, in the very language. In Arabic script, as in Hebrew, no vowels are set down, only consonants... Until life is literally breathed into them, Arabic and Hebrew words on the page have no particular meaning...Indeed, until then they are not words but only potential words, a chaotic possibility of meanings. It is as if the scripts of these languages, marshaling their bare consonants across the page, hold within them vast spaces where meanings exist in a condition of whirling potentiality until the moment that one is singled out and uttered. And so by their very scripts, Hebrew and Arabic seem to announce the primacy of the spoken, living word; they announce that meaning can only be here and now. Here and now in this body, this breath (*nafas*), this self (*nafs*) encounters the word, gives it life (Ahmed, 2000, pp. 95-96).

'Here and now in this body'; this is the refrain of the Arab women of somatic metaphor, of proverb, of song. 'Here and now in this body,' they seem to say, we will take this breath and this self and 'encounter the word,' and 'give it life'.

In these pages, we have seen many ways in which Arab women in the Middle East – mothers and others – use language to convey their experiences of themselves and their societies. These women, enculturated in a 'holistic' environment (Dwairy, 1998), are disinclined to bifurcate their minds and their bodies, leaning instead toward the sort of monism that until a very few years ago was the stuff of life for all, East and West alike. Thus, in a review of Furst's *Idioms of Distress: Psychosomatic Disorders in Medical and Imaginative Literature*, Robert Nye (2005) tells us that the author believes that:

> ...a holistic account of the mind/body relationship has been irresistible to generations of writers...not just as a metaphorical adornment in their work,

but as an inescapable aspect of their observations of the lived experience (Nye, 2005, p. 244).

Nye further writes that Furst:

> ...suggests that literary treatments of these conditions [psychosomatic symptoms and disorders] permit us to see them develop in the broadest possible social and psychological setting, where the ideals, expectations, and judgments of society burden individuals with disciplines that are unbearably harsh but so exigent that resistance to them takes unconscious bodily form. Where words and arguments fail, the body speaks its suffering symptomatically (Nye, 2005, p. 245).

Here, we have reviewed some of the pressing disciplines imposed upon women throughout the world, and upon Arab/Islamic women in the Middle East particularly. Most notably, we have seen from different standpoints the ideal of allegiance to family and community, so central to sociocentric societies such as the Arab one. We have noted the support such societies grant to members who act in accordance with their rules, and the censure they mete out to those who do not. So too, the powerful communitarian thrust in the region was revealed in the traditional treatment modalities, emphasizing group participation and ritual. The entire notion of spirit possession, illustrated, for instance, in the *zar* ceremony, was discussed as an idiom of distress that accommodates some important emotional and cultural needs of the group in the Arab region. And, as van Duijl, Nijenhuis, Komproe, Hajo, Gernaat, and de Jong (2010) stress in their work on possession among trauma survivors in Uganda,

> ...spirit possession...in itself is not pathological. Only when this, as an attribution or as a dissociative presentation, is causing clinically significant distress...can it be classified as a disorder (p. 394).

Recognizing, then, that this sociocentric system is a fundament of Arab life, yet not impenetrable, we reviewed a number of psychotherapeutic approaches for treating women in the Arab region. Befitting the non-egocentric nature of their culture, these techniques highlight family work, with culturally demanded respect granted to the male authority figure. Directive, goal-oriented treatment is advised often, and metaphor therapies are by their nature conducive to work with individuals who are inclined to speak in metaphoric, poetic terms when expressing emotional pain. Mindfulness therapies are being investigated for efficacy with somatic symptom disorder, and some preliminary studies using a longitudinal design and controlled methods point to possible further directions for the treatment of Arab women.

Crucially, we have proposed a tripartite mental health treatment program for Arab women in the Middle East; this is based on a major research study, which was presented in chapter seven. The three essential elements of this model, which we call 'Wrap-Around Resilience,' are: (1) A biomedical approach that flexibly and consistently makes use of practitioners who understand, and also may employ, traditional intervention techniques; (2) A primary-care treatment base that is trained to identify and manage the gamut of biopsychosocial needs attendant to the somatic complaints of Arab women in the Arab region; and (3) a targeted outreach effort toward divorced Arab women, who have been shown to be at heightened risk for emotional, social and economic distress. Here, as well, we suggest taking up family policy expert Karen Bogenschneider's idea of a 'family impact lens' (2012, cited in Lamanna, Riedman and Stewart, 2014, p. 22). Employing such a tool, we would evaluate mental health policy-making for Arab women in the MENA region from the patient's primary point of view: how it impacts on her family: natal, marital, and extended. In this manner, a macro- as well as micro-planning perspective could be implemented in which the sociocentric nature of Arab society is taken properly into account. These three components would be built around the 'ecological resilience' strategies that are now being developed from their currently emergent form (Ungar, 2013).

Overall, our proposed program demonstrates a strong affinity with global directions in health provision. As noted by the Director-General of the WHO, in presenting its Traditional Medicine Strategy 2014-2023:

> T&CM [traditional medicine and non-conventional medicine] is an important and often underestimated part of health care. T&CM is found in almost every country in the world and the demand for its services is increasing (Chan, 2014, p. 7).

Concluding this section of the chapter, we note that no one culture has a monopoly on best-living practices, on the 'proper' way-to-be in the world. Below, some renowned scholars of Islam elaborate on this theme.

The 'Social Life' of Muslim Women's Rights

In a paper titled *The Active Social Life of 'Muslim Women's Rights'* (2012) and then in a related volume, Lila Abu-Lughod makes an ethnographic 'plea' for investigating how the 'women's rights industry creates careers, channels funds, inspires commitments, gives credibility to new actors, creates and disrupts social networks, and legitimizes intellectual and political frameworks and ideals' (p. 33). In sum, Abu-Lughod proposes that attention be paid to what gets achieved and who achieves it by pursuing Arab women's rights, and especially a construction of those rights as 'universal.' Most of all, she seeks to encourage an examination of how the 'rallying cry' of Muslim women's rights works to 'save Muslim women from their cultures...' (2012, p. 16). Among the same Awlad 'Ali women we know from the *ghinnassa*, the author determined that:

> ...the framework and the projects of 'Muslim women's rights' do not begin to exhaust these women's conceptions of rights and their experiences of trying to assert them in everyday life (Abu-Lughod, 2012, p. 34).

Indeed, one might venture that the *ghinnassa* serve as an alternative means for these women to assert their rights, at least in Leila Ahmed's sense of:

> Meaning always only here and now, in this body, for this person. Truth always only here and now, for this body, this person (Ahmed, 2000, p. 96).

The truth 'for this body, this person' also seems an apt way of understanding the Bedouin women of the Negev, whose lived experience of divorce, for example, was suffused with somatic signs of distress.

In an earlier paper, Ahmed (1982) deftly disposed of the longstanding western notion that women's *ways of being* in the Arab region are inherently disrespectful of and damaging to them. Choosing the 'harem' or separate female space as her example (long focused on 'with fascination and loathing' by western males), the author clarified that as much as the term could apply to 'a system that permits males sexual access to more than one female' (p. 524), it can be thought of:

> ...with just as much accuracy, as a system whereby the female relatives of a man – wives, sisters, mother, aunts, daughters – share...their time and their living space, and...which enables women to have frequent and easy access to

> other women in their community... (Ahmed, 1982, p. 524).

Notably, Ahmed is no apologist for patriarchy. Quite the contrary. Nonetheless, the author, a noted scholar of Islamic studies at the Harvard University School of Divinity, tells in her autobiography of having been raised in a sort of harem, and as having rather liked it.

In this last section of the chapter, and the final one of the book, we arrive at a sense of limitation, of humility in the face of the radical complexity of the human condition. The three instances I shall offer here pertain to three different but interrelated points of impossibility. First, we will consider what Kirmayer (2008) has termed 'the limits of clinical empathy in situations of radical otherness' (p. 457). As a second example, we will take up Abu-Lughod's (2013) reservations regarding the pursuance of universal rights for the entire world, and specifically for the women of the world. We will conclude with Leighton and colleagues' concerns for the nature of the cultural psychiatry project, and its natural bounds.

In a recent paper that engages with the challenges of alterity and empathy in the clinical relationship, Kirmayer (2008) goes just about as far as he can go in seeking the terms of a truly empathetic psychotherapeutic stance. He begins with a fairly standard description of empathy: 'the willingness to meet, engage, and be moved by the other – whether that other is an esthetic object or a person' (p. 458). The author then takes us on a fascinating journey, creating a veritable travelogue of the different constructions of therapeutic empathy, finally arriving at 'the failure, fracture, or even radical impossibility of empathy' (p. 470). And it is here that our guide pauses, because it is here that he wishes for us to take in the view. When Kirmayer begins again, it is with the sobering notion that:

> ,,,cultural and psychological (mis)appropriation, narcissism, collusion, and submission to the powerful can create the illusion of empathy where something radically different is at play: the effacement or annihilation of the other...(Kirmayer, 2008, p. 470).

Nonetheless, despair is not in order:

> In place of the false fusion of empathic understanding, a new possibility of knowing through dialogue can be built on the moment of resistance, rupture, and difference...the process of acknowledging failures of empathy then constitutes the real achievement of the effort to encounter the other – an encounter that is always partial, conditional, transient, and fragile. Each act of encounter works toward constituting a social world that can tolerate, contain

> and even foster our essential difference (Kirmayer, 2008, p. 471).
>
> 'Essential difference' drives Abu-Lughod. She proposes an unalterable, impossible-to-elide difference among individuals in which some women
>
> ...might be called to personhood, so to speak, in different languages (Abu-Lughod, 2013, p. 43).

Thus, after affirming the basic goodness of seeking justice and rights for women, the author asks,

> ...but can we accept that there might be different ideas of about justice, and that different women might want, or even choose, different futures from ones that we envision as best? (Abu-Lughod, 2013, p. 43).

Following Kirmayer above, we might suggest that the 'sensationalist' and otherwise agenda-driven hunts for the 'rights of Muslim women' to which Abu-Lughod vigorously points are instances of a 'false fusion of empathetic understanding,' implying an 'effacement of the other' rather than true encounter. The roiling international veil controversy serves as an excellent example of a cultural misappropriation: as Ahmed (2011) has laid out in exacting historical detail, the world's 'women of cover' seem to evince little interest in being stripped of their scarves. Fine intentions aside, then, what we can determine as 'right' for any other person is circumscribed by the existential truth of each person's otherness.

And so we come to our final point of human possibility. Leighton, the father of cultural psychiatry, admitted:

> Thus our men and women, each by each, and taken all together as a community, are left so many dangling questions. But then, life dangles; only conundrums have answers. Life flows in its arcs and streamers of multicolors, but it is not pulled together for us, it is not explained, and neither misery nor happiness are guaranteed. Lines are fixed only in death, madness, and fiction (Leighton, 1959, p. 227).

In Leighton's humble words we hear the tone of truth. While we have made an honest effort in these pages to limn the emotional lives of Arab women in the Middle East, taking into account best practices of cultural psychiatry in its thus-far most developed, globally responsive guise, we are acutely aware of the gaps, the empty spaces, the 'dangling questions.' But, like Kirmayer and Abu-Lughod above, Leighton leaves us finally with a different sense, a sense of purpose for refinement, for hope:

> It is by search and research that we can…secure the means to …rescue others and to rescue ourselves (1959, p. 392).

Now, rescue is a loaded word. Indeed, we have learned, or are beginning to learn, that the 'rescue' (or, in Abu-Lughod's terms, 'saving') of others is fraught with complication. Rather, we now know to strive for (as difficult as that is to do) a sharp analysis of the nature of complex interrelations, as well as a recognition of our political and ideological premises. But Leighton does not stop at the expected moment: he brings us all into the picture. And it is here that we can feel on firmer footing – to 'search and research,' that is, to plumb our personal and communal depths for the ways and means to rescue our own selves and communities from the pain and injustice that we meet on a moment-to-moment basis. That, following Leighton, is 'the issue, the solution, the object' (1959, p. 392).

References

Aarts, P., (2012). *Saudi Arabia: Between Conservatism, Accommodation and Reform.* Netherlands Institute of International Relations.

Abbo, C., Ekblad, S., Waako, P., Okello, E., Muhwezi, W., Musis, S. (2008). Psychological distress and associated factors among the attendees of traditional healing practices in Jinja and Iganga districts, Eastern Uganda: A cross-sectional study. *International Journal of Mental Health Systems,* 2(1), 16.

Abdel-Khalek, Ahmed M.; Alansari, Bader M. (2004). Gender Differences in Anxiety among Undergraduates from Ten Arab Countries. *Social Behavior and Personality: An International Journal,* 32(7).

Abrahams, R.D. (1968a). Introductory remarks to a rhetorical theory of folklore. *Journal of American Folklore, 81,* 143-157.

Abu-Baker, K. (2005). The impact of social values on the psychology of gender among Arab couples: A view from psychotherapy. *Israeli Journal of Relational Science,* 42(2), 106-115.

Abu-Lughod, L. (1985). A community of secrets: the separate world of Bedouin women. *Journal of Women in Culture and Society, 10,* 637-657.

Abu-Lughod, L. (1985). *Veiled Sentiments.* Berkeley & Los Angeles, London: University of California Press.

Abu-Lughod, L. (2010). The active social life of 'Muslim women's rights': A plea for ethnography, not polemic, with cases from Egypt and Palestine. *Journal of Middle East Women's Studies,* 6(1), 1-45.

Abu-Lugod, L. (2013). *Do Muslim Women Need Saving?* Cambridge, MA & London, England: Harvard University Press.

Abu-Odeh L. (1996) Crimes of honor and the construction of gender in Arab societies. In M. Yamani (Ed.), *Feminism and Islam: Legal and Literary Perspectives,* New York, NY: University Press.

Abu Rabia-Queder, S. (2007). Permission to rebel: Arab Bedouin women's changing negotiation of social roles. *Feminist Studies,* 33(1), 161-187.

Afifi, M. and von Bothmer, M. (20007). Egyptian women's attitudes and beliefs aboutfemale genital cutting and its association with childhood maltreatment *Nursing and Health Sciences, 9,* 70–276.

Ahmad, D. (2009). Not Yet Beyond the Veil: Muslim Women in American Popular Literature. *Social Text, 27*(2) 99, 105-131.

Ahmed, K.,Bhugra, D. (2007). Depression across ethnic minority cultures: diagnostic issues. *World Cultural Psychiatry Research Review,* 47-56.

Ahmed, L., (1982). Western ethnocentrism and perceptions of the harem. *Feminist Studies,* 8(3), 521-534.

Ahmed, L. (1985). Women and the advent of Islam. *Journal of Women in Culture and Society, 11*(4), 665-691.

Ahmed, L. (1989). Arab culture and writing women's bodies. *Feminist Issues*, 41-54.

Ahmed, L. (1999). *A border passage: from Cairo to America – a woman's journey.* New York: Penguin Group.

Ahmed, L., (2000). The Women of Islam. *Transition, 9*(3), 78-95.

Ahmed, L., (2011). *Quiet Revolution: The Veil's Resurgence.* USA: Yale University Press.

Adeponle, A., Whitley, R., Kirmayer, L. (2012). Cultural contexts and constructions of recovery. In A. Rudnick (Ed.), *Recovery of people with mental illness: Philosophical and related perspectives* (pp.109-132). New York, NY: Oxford University Press.

Akilova, M.Y. and Marti, Y.M.,(2014). What is the Effect of Women's Financial Empowerment on Intimate Partner Violence in Jordan? *Glob Soc Welf.* doi: 10.1007/s40609-014-0005-x

Albright, W.F. (1940). Islam and the religions of the ancient Orient. *The Journal of the American Oriental Society, 60*, 283-286.

Al-Adawi, S. Dorvlo, A.S., Al-Ismaily, S.S., Al-Ghafry, D.A. Al-Noobi, B.Z., Al-Salmi, A., Burke, D.T., Shah, M.K., Ghassany, H., & Chand, S.P. (2002). Perceptions and attitude towards mental illness in Oman. *International Journal of Social Psychiatry, 48*(4), 305-315.

Al-Antiel, F. (1978). *Between the folklore and public culture* [in Arabic]. Cairo: Al-Hiah Al-Massriah Llketab.

Al-Ashquar, U.S. (2005). *The world of the Jinn and devils.* International Islamic Publishing House.

Al-Haj, M. (1987) *Social Change and Family Processes: Arab Communities in Shefar-A'm.* London: Westview Press.

Al-Issa, I. (Ed.) (1995). *Handbook of Culture and Mental Illness: An International Perspective.* Madison, Connecticut: International Universities Press, Inc.

Al-Issa, I. (Ed.) (2000). *Al-Junun: Mental illness in the Islamic world.* Madison, Connecticut: International Universities Press, Inc.

Al-Krenawi, A. (1996). Group work with Bedouin widows of the Negev in a medical clinic. *Affilia: Journal of Women and Social Work, 11(3)*, 303-318.

Al-Krenawi, A. (1998a). Family therapy with a multiparental/multispousal family. *Family Process, 37(1)*, 65-81.

Al-Krenawi, A. (1998b). Reconciling western treatment and traditional healing: A social worker walks with the wind. *Reflections: Narrative of Professional Helping, 4*(3), 6-21.

Al-Krenawi, A. (1999a). Explanation of mental health symptoms by the Bedouin-Arabs of the Negev. *International Journal of Social Psychiatry, 45*(1), 56-64.

Al-Krenawi, A. (1999b). Integrating cultural rituals into family therapy: A case study with a Bedouin-Arab patient in Israel. *Journal of family Psychotherapy, 10*(1).

Al-Krenawi, A. (2002). Mental health service utilization among the Arabs in Israel. *Social work in health care,* 35(1-2), 577-589.

Al-Krenawi, A. & Graham, J.R. (1996). Social work practice and traditional healing rituals among the Bedouin of the Negev. *International Social Work, 39,* 177-188.

Al-Krenawi, A. & Graham, J.R. (1997a). Social work and blood vengeance: The Bedouin-Arab case. *British Journal of Social Work, 27,* 515-528.

Al-Krenawi, A. & Graham, J.R. (1997b). Nebi-Musa: A therapeutic community for drug addicts in a Muslim context. *Transcultural Psychiatry, 34(3),* 377-391.

Al-Krenawi, A. & Graham, J.R. (1997c). Spirit possession and exorcism: The integration of modern and traditional mental health care systems in the treatment of a Bedouin patient. *Clinical Social Work Journal, 25,* 211-222.

Al-Krenawi, A., & Graham, J. R. (1998). Divorce among Muslim Arab women in Israel. *Journal of Divorce and Remarriage, 29(3/4),* 103-119.

Al-Krenawi, A. & Graham, J.R. (1999). Social work practice and female genital mutilation. *Social Development Issue, 21(1),* 29-36.

Al-Krenawi, A., & Graham, J. R. (2000). Culturally-sensitive social work practice with Arab clients in mental health settings. *Health & Social Work,* 25(1), 9-22.

Al-Krenawi, A., & Graham, J.R. (2001). The cultural mediator: Bridging the gap between a non-western community and professional social work practice. *British Journal of Social Workers, 31,* 665-685.

Al-Krenawi, A., & Graham, J.R. (2004). Somatization among Bedouin-Arab women. *Journal of Divorce and Remarriage,* 42(1-2), 131-143, doi:10.1300/ JO87v42n01 06

Al-Krenawi, A., Graham, J. R., & Al-Krenawi, S. (1997). Social work practice with polygamous families. *Child and Adolescent Social Work Journal,* 25(6), 445-458

Al-Krenawi, A., Graham, .J.R., & Kandah, J. (2000). Gendered utilization differences of mental health services in Jordan. *Community Mental Health Journal,* 36(5), 501-511.

Al-Krenawi, A., Graham, J. R., & Slonim-Nevo, V. (2002). Mental health aspects of Arab adolescents of polygamous/monogamous families. *The Journal of Social Psychology.* 142 (4), 446-460.

Al-Krenawi, A., & Wiesel-Lev, R. (1999). Attitudes toward and perceived psychosocial impact of female circumcision as practiced among the Bedouin-Arabs of the Negev. *Family Processes,* 38, 431-443.

Al-Mutairi N., Al-Farag S, Al-Mutairi A, Al-Shiltawy M. (2010). Comorbidities associated with psoriasis: an experience from the Middle East. *The Journal of Dermatology.* 37(2), 146-55. doi: 10.1111/j.1346-8138.2009.00777.x.

Al-Nsour, M., Khawaja, M., Al-Kayyali, G. (2009). Domestic violence against women in Jordan: Evidence from health clinics. *Journal of Family Violence.* doi: 10.1007/s1089-009-9255-2

Al-Sadawi, N. (1985). Growing up female in Egypt. In E.W. Feranea (Ed.), *Women and the family in the Middle East:N voices of change.* (pp. 111-120). Austin: University of Texas Press.

Ameen, A.K.I. 2005. *The jinn and human sickness: remedies in the light of the Quran and Sunnah. Riyadh: Darussalam.*

American Psychiatric Association (2013). *Diagnostic and Statistical Manual of Mental Disorders: DSM-5.* Washington, DC: AMA.

Amin, Hamdi and Abou-Saleh (2001). Depression in the Arab world. In Okasha & Maj (Eds.), *Images in Psychiatry: An Arab Perspective* (pp. 89-122). Cairo: World Psychiatric Association.

Amering, M. (2010). Trialog—an exercise in communication between consumers, carers and professional mental health workers beyond role stereotypes. *International Journal of Integrated Care, 10*(5).

Ammar, N.H. (2007). Wife battery in Islam. *Violence Against Women, 13*(5), 516-526.

Antonovsky, A. (1993). The structure and properties of the sense of coherence scale. *Social Science and Medicine, 36*(2), 725-733.

Antonovsky, A. (1987). *Unraveling the mystery of health: how people manage stress and stay well.* San Francisco: Jossey-Bass.

Asali, A., Khamaysi, N., Aburabia, Y., Letzer, S., Halihal, B., Sadovsky, M., ... & Belmaker, R. H. (1995). Ritual female genital surgery among Bedouin in Israel. *Archives of Sexual Behavior, 24*(5), 571-575.

Aslan, R. (2013). Women in the Workforce in the Arab World. *Insight:*

Atallah, D. (2013, December 21). The Story of a West Bank Honour Killing. *The Jerusalem Post.*

Aviera, A. (1996). 'Dichos' therapy group: A therapeutic use of Spanish language proverbs with hospitalized Spanish-speaking psychiatric patients. *Cultural Diversity and Mental Health, 2*(2), 73-87.

Ayonrinde, A.O. (1977). Heat in the head or body – a semantic confusion? *African Journal of Psychiatry, 1,* 59-63.

Ballantyne, P.J. (1999) The social determinants of health: a contribution to the analysis of gender differences in health and illness. *Scand J Public Health 27,* 290–295.

Barakat, H. (1985). The Arab family and the challenge of social transformation. In E.W. Fernea (Ed.), *Women and the family in the Middle East: New voices of change* (pp. 27-48). Austin: University of Texas Press.

Barakat, H. (1993). *The Arab world: Society, culture, and state.* Los Angeles: University of California Press.

Barkow, J. H. (2006). Alexander Leighton and the evolutionary perspective. *Transcultural psychiatry, 43*(1), 45-55.

Barsky, A.J. (2014). Assessing somatic symptoms in clinical practice. *Journal of the American Medical Association, 174*(3), 407-408.

Barsky, A.J., Ahern, D.K., Bauer, M.R., Nolido, N., Orav, J. (2012). A randomized trial of treatments for high-utilizing somatising patients. *Journal of General Internal Medicine, 28*(11), 1396-404.

Barsky, A.J. & Klerman, G.L. (1983). Overview: hypochondriasis, bodily complaints, and somatic styles. *The American Journal of Psychiatry, 140,* 273-283.

Bazzoui, W. (1970) Affective Disorders in Iraq. *British Journal of Psychiatry, 112*(489), 827-832.

Beck, L. & Keddie, N. (1978). *Women in the Muslim World,* Cambridge, MA and London, England: Harvard University Press.

Becker, S.M. (2004). Detection of somatization and depression in primary care in Saudi Arabia. *Social Psychiatry and Psychiatric Epidemiology,*39(12), 962-6.

Beeble, M. L., & Salem, D. A. (2009). Understanding the phases of recovery from serious mental illness: the roles of referent and expert power in a mutual-help setting. *Journal of Community Psychology, 37*(2), 249-267.

Beiser, M. (2003). Why should researchers care about culture? *Canadian Journal of Psychiatry, 48*(3), 154-159.

Bellin, E., (2004) The Robustness of Authoritarianism in the Middle East: Exceptionalism in Comparative. *Comparative Politics,* 36(2), 139-157.

Ben-David, Y. (July, 1999) *The Bedouin in Israel.* Retrieved from http://www.mfa.gov.il/mfa/mfa-archive/1999/pages/the%20bedouin%20in%20israel.aspx

Bener, A., Al-Kazaz, M., Ftouni, D., Al-Harthy, M., Dafeeah, E.E. (2013). Diagnostic overlap of depressive, anxiety, stress and somatoform disorders in primary care. *Asia-Pacific Psychiatry,* 5, E29-E38.

Bener A, Burgut FT, Ghuloum S and Sheikh J. (2011). *A Study of Postpartum Depression in a Fast Developing Country: Prevalence and Related Factors.* Gold Coast, Australia: The 12th International Mental Health Conference: Personality Disorders: Out of the Darkness.

Berque, J. (1964). *The Arabs: Their History & Future.* London: Faber & Faber.

Bhugra, D., Mastrogianni, A. (2004). Globalisation and mental disorders. Overview with relation to depression. *Br J Psychiatry. 184,* 10-20.

Blue I, Ducci ME, and Jaswal S. (1995). The mental health of low income urban women. In T. Harpham and I. Blue (Eds.), *Urbanisation and Mental Health in Developing Countries* (pp. 75–102). Aldershot: Avebury.

Bodhi, B. (2000). *A comprehensive manual of Adhidhamma.* Seattle: BPS Paariyatti.

Bogenschneider, K. (2014). *Family Policy Matters: How Policymaking Affects Families and What Professionals Can Do.* New York, NY: Routledge.

Boy, A., Kulczycki, A. (2008). What we know about intimate partner violence in the Middle East and North Africa. *Violence Against Women, 14*(1), 53-70.

Braddy, C.M., Files, J.A. (2007).Female genital mutilation: cultural awareness and clinical considerations. *J. Midwifery Womens Health,* 52, 158–163.

Brandsma, L. (2007). Eating Disorders across the Life Span. In V. Malatesta (Ed.), Mental Health Issues of Older Women: A Comprehensive Review for Health Care Professionals (pp. 155-172). Binghamton, NY: Haworth Press.

Breaking Israel News. (2013, December 13). Rising Trend of Palestinian 'Honor Killings'. Retrieved from http://www.breakingisraelnews.com/7967/rising-trend-palestinian-honor-killings/#P8RDJse1GAC3hEYd.99

Brhoom, M. (1987). The phenomenon of divorce in Jordan (in Arabic). *Dirasat, 13*(12), 189-205.

Bridges, K., Goldberg, D., Evans, B. & Sharpe, T. (1991). Determinants of somatization in primary care. *Psychological Medicine, 21,* 478-483.

Bronfenbrenner, U. (1979). *The ecology of human development: Experiments by nature and design.* Cambridge, MA: Harvard University Press.

Buist-Bouwman, M.A., De Graaf, R., Vollebergh, W.A., Alonso, J., Bruffaerts, R, Ormel, J., (2006). Functional disability of mental disorders and comparison with physical disorders: a study among the general population of six European countries. *Acta Psychiatr Scand, 113*(6), 492–500.

Burke TK and Reardon CD. (1988). *Abortion Trauma and Child Abuse.* PA: Post Abortion Review.

Centers for Disease Control and Prevention (2013). *Mental health surveillance among children – United States, 2005—2011,* 1-35.

Chaleby, K., Al-Haj, O., & Bukhari, H. (1989). Divorced Saudi women: A study of a psychiatric outpatient population. *Arab Journal of Psychiatry, 1*(1), 43-48.

Chesler, P. (2009). Are honor killings simply domestic violence? *The Middle East Quarterly,* 61-69.

Chaudhry, A. (2014). *Domestic Violence and the Islamic Tradition.* USA: Oxford University Press.

Chisholm, D., Flisher, A.J., Lund, C., Patel, V., Saxena, S., Thornicroft, G., Tomlinson, M. (2007). Scale up services for mental disorders: a call for action. *Lancet, 370,* 1241–52.

Christodoulou,G.N. (2012) Depression as caused by the economic crisis. In *Depression, a global crisis.* World Federation for Mental Health.

Chung, R.C.-Y. (2006). Human Trafficking for Sexual Exploitation: Psychological & Cultural Impacts. *Global Studies Review,* 2(3).

Clifton-Soderstrom, M. (2003). Levinas and the patient as other: The ethical foundation of medicine. *Journal of Medicine and Philosophy, 28*(3), 448-460.

Clarke, D.M., Piterman, L., Byrne, C.J. & Austin, D.W. (2008).Somatic symptoms, hypochondriasis and psychological distress: a study of somatization in

Australian general practice. *MJA, 189*(10), 560-563.

Cohen, O, and Savaya, R. (1997). Broken glass: The divorced woman in Moslem Arab society in Israel. *Family process. 36*(3), 225-245.

Costa , P. T. &. McCrae Jr., R. R. (1985). The NEO Personality Inventory manual. Odessa, FL: Psychological Assessment Resources.

Department of Health and Human Services Centers for Disease Control and Prevention (2003). *Costs of Intimate Partner Violence Against Women in the United States.* Atlanta, Georgia.

Creed, F.H., Davies, I., Jackson, J., Littlewood, A., Cheew-Graham, C., Tomenson, B., Macfarlane, G., Barsky, A., Katon, W, McBeth, J. The epidemiology of multiple somatic symptoms. *Journal of Psychosomatic Research, 72,* 311-317.

Danaci, A.E., Dinç, G., Deveci,A., Seyfe Şen, F., İçelli, I. (2002). Postnatal depression in Turkey: epidemiological and cultural aspects. *Social Psychiatry and Psychiatric Epidemiology, 37*(3), 125-129.

Davis, D.M. & Hayes, J.A. (2011). What are the benefits of mindfulness? A practice review of psychotherapy-related research. *Psychotherapy, 48*(2), 198-208.

Democratic Control of Armed Forces (DCAF). (2005). *Women in an Insecure World.* Geneva: Vlachovà, M. and Biason, L.

De Jong, J.T., Reis, R. (2010). Kiyang-yang, a West-African postwar idiom of distress, *Cultural Medical Psychiatry, 34,* 301-321.

Deen, T. (2014, March 16). Women Still Walk Two Steps Behind in Arab World. *Inter Press Service.*

Demyttenaere, K., Bruffaerts, R., Posada-Villa, J., Gasquet, I., Kovess, V., Lepine, J.P., Angermeyer, M.C., Bernert S, de Girolamo G, Morosini P, Polidori G, Kikkawa T, Kawakami N, Ono Y, Takeshima T, Uda H, Karam EG, Fayyad JA, Karam AN, Mneimneh ZN, Medina-Mora ME, Borges G, Lara C, de Graaf R, Ormel J, Gureje O, Shen Y, Huang Y, Zhang M, Alonso J, Haro JM, Vilagut G, Bromet EJ, Gluzman S, Webb C, Kessler RC, Merikangas KR, Anthony JC, Von Korff MR, Wang PS, Brugha TS, Aguilar-Gaxiola S, Lee S, Heeringa S, Pennell BE, Zaslavsky AM, Ustun TB, Chatterji S. (2004). Prevalence, severity, and unmet need for treatment of mental disorders in the World Health Organization World Mental Health Surveys. *JAMA. 291,* 2581–2590.

Desjarlais R., Eisenberg, L., Good, B. Kleinman, A. (1996). (Eds.), *World Mental Health: Problems and Priorities in Low-Income Countries.* New York: Oxford University Press.

Derogatis, L.R. (1992). *SCL-90-R manual: administration, scoring and procedures.* Baltimore, MD: Clinical Psychometric Research.

Derogatis, L.R. (1977). *SCL-90-R administration, scoring and procedure manual for R (revised) version.* Baltimore: John Hopkins University School of Medicine.

Dickerson, F.B. (2007). Women, aging and schizophrenia. In V. Malatesta (Ed.), *Mental Health Issues of Older Women: A Comprehensive Review for Health Care Professionals* (pp. 49-62). Binghamton, NY: Haworth Press.

Didonna, F. (Ed.). (2009). *Clinical handbook of mindfulness*. New York: Springer.

Diener, E., Emmons, R.A., Larsen, R.J., & Griffin, S. (1985). The satisfaction with life scale. *Journal of Personality Assessment, 49*, 71-75.

Dimsdale, J.E., Creed, F. Escobar, J., Sharpe, M. Wulsin, L., Barsky, A., Lee, S., Irwin, M.R., Levenson, J. (2013). Somatic symptom disorder: An important change in DSM. *Journal of Psychosomatic Research, 75*, 223-228.

Diop-Sidibe, N., Campbell, J. C. & Becker, S. (2006). Domestic violence against women in Egypt—wife beating and health outcomes. *Social Science & Medicine*, 62, 1260-1277. http://dx.doi.org/10.1016/j.socscimed.2005.07.022

Douki, S. Ben Zineb, S., Nacef, F., Halbreich, U. (2007). Women's mental health in the Muslim world: Cultural, religious, and social issues. *Journal of Affective Disorders, 102*, 177-189.

Drieskins, B. (2008). *Living with Djinns: Understanding and dealing with the invisible in Cairo*. London, UK: Saqi Books.

Dura-Vila, G. Hodes, M. (2012). Cross-cultural study of idioms of distress among Spanish nationals and Hispanic American migrants: *susto, nervios* and *ataque de nervios. Social Psychiatry Psychiatric Epidemiology, 47*, 1627-1637.

Dwairy, M. A. (1998). *Cross-Cultural Counseling: The Arab-Palestinian Case*. New York: Haworth Press.

Eisner, M. & Ghuneim, L. (2013). Honor Killing Attitudes Amongst Adolescents in Amman, Jordan. *Aggressive Behavior*, 9999, pp. 1–13.

Elgousi, H.S. (2011). Female genital mutilation between culture and religion: The case of Egypt. In M. Ennaji and F. Sadiqi (Eds.), *Gender and Violence in the Middle East*. UCLA Center for Middle East Development (CMED) series: Routledge.

Elshahawi, H., Hussein, H., Mobarak, M., Allam, M., Enas A. (2011). Depression comorbidity in patients with chronic hepatitis C and its possible relation to treatment outcome. *Middle East Current Psychiatry*, 18(1), 23–28. doi: 10.1097/01.XME.0000392845.09854.6f

El-Islam, M.F. (1982). Arabic cultural psychiatry. *Transcultural Psychiatric Research Review, 19*, 5-24.

El-Islam, M.F. (1982b). Rehabilitation of schizophrenics by the extended family. *Acta Psychiatrica Scandinavica, 65*, 112-119.

El-Islam, M. F., Moussa, M. A. A., Malasi, T. H., Suleiman, M. A., & Mirza, I. A. (1988). Assessment of depression in Kuwait by principal component analysis. *Journal of affective disorders, 14*(2), 109-114.

El-Islam M. F. (1989). Collaboration With Families For Rehabilitation of Schizophrenic Patients and the Concept of Expressed Emotion. *Acta Psychiatrica Scandinavica, 79*, 303-307.

El-Islam, M.F. (1983). Cultural change and intergenerational relationship in Arabian families. *International Journal of Family Psychiatry, 4*(4), 321-329.

El-Islam, M.F. (2008). Arab culture and mental health care. *Transcultural Psychiatry, 45*(4), 671-682. doi: 10.1177/1363461508100788

El-Saadani, S. (2006). Divorce in the Arab region: Current levels, trends and features. Retrieved from www.infostat.sk/vdc/epc2006/papers/epc2006s60046.pdf

El-Shenawi, E. (2011). Poking at the Beast: How much is the Arab world worth? *Al-Arabya News*. Retrieved from http://english.alarabiya.net/articles/2011/05/05/147980.htm

El-Rufaie, O.E.F., Al-Sabosy, M.M.A., Bener, A. & Abuzeid, M.S.O. (1999). Somatized Mental Disorder Among Primary Care Arab Patients: I. Prevalence and Clinical and Sociodemographic Characteristics. *Journal of Psychosomatic Research, 46*(6), 549-555.

Ennaji M., and Sadiqi, F. (Eds.). (2011). *Gender and Violence in the Middle East.* UCLA Center for Middle East Development (CMED) series): Routledge.

Epstein, E.E., Fishcher-Elber, K.,& Al-Otaiba, Z. (2007). Women, Aging and Alcohol Use disorders. In V. Maltesta (Ed.), Mental Health Issues of Older Women: A Comprehensive Review for Health Care Professionals (pp. 31-48). Binghamton, NY: Haworth Press.

Epstein, N.B., Baldwin, M.N. & Bishop, D.S. (1983). The McMaster Family Assessment Device. *Journal of Marital and Family Therapy, 9,* 171-180.

Erikson, E.H. (1963). *Childhood and society* (2nd ed.). New York: Norton.

Escobar, J.L., Burnan, A., Karno, M., Forsythe, A. & Golding, J.M. (1987). Somatization in the community. *Archives of general psychiatry, 44,* 713-718.

Escobar, J.L., Ribio-Stipec, M. Canino, G., Karno, M. (1989). Somatic Symptom Index (SSI): a new and abridged somatization construct. *Journal of Nervous and Mental Disease, 177,* 140-146.

Fabrega, H. (1991). The culture and history of psychiatric stigma in early modern and modern Western societies: A review of recent literature. *Comprehensive Psychiatry, 32(2),* 97-119.

Faksh, M.A. (1997). Review of Martin Kramer 'Arab Awakening and Islamic Revival: The Politics of Ideas in the Middle East. *The Review of Politics, 59,* 633-636. doi:10.1017/S0034670500027856

Faramarzi, M., Esmailzadeh, S., & Mosavi, S. (2005). Prevalence and determinants of intimate partner violence in Babol City, Islamic Republic of Iran. *Eastern Mediterranean Health Journal, 11,* 870–79.

Feldner, Y. (2000). 'Honor' Murders – Why the perps get off easy. *Middle East Quarterly,* 41-50.

Fernandez, J.V. (1977). The performance of ritual metaphors In J.D. Sapir & I.C.

Crocker (Eds.), *The social use of metaphors: Essays on the anthropology of the rhetoric*. Philadelphia: University of Pennsylvania Press.

Fisch, R. Weakland, J.H. and Segal, L. (1992). *The tactics of change: Doing therapy briefly*. San Francisco: Jossey-Bass.

Fjorback, L.O., Arendt, M., Ornbol, E., Walach, H., Rehfeld, E., Schroder, A. & Fink, P. (2012). Mindfulness therapy for somatization disorder and unctional somatic syndromes – randomized trial with one-year follow-up. *Journal of Psychosomatic Research, 74*(1), 31-40.

Fox, M. (2014, September 16). The Horror of Honor Killing: In America and Around the World. *The Huffington Post.*

Franco, M. (2007). Post Traumatic Stress Disorder and Older Women. In V. Malatesta (Ed.), *Mental Health Issues of Older Women: A Comprehensive Review for Health Care Professionals* (pp. 103-118). Binghamton, NY: The Haworth Press.

Freund, C. (2013).*The surprising rates of depression among MENA's women*. The World Bank.

Galvan, R.A. & Teschner, R.V. (1985). *El diccionario del Espanol Chicano* [The dictionary of Chicano Spanish]. Lincolnwood, IL: National Textbook Company.

García-Moreno, C., Jansen, H.A.F.M., Ellsberg, M., Heise, and L.,Watts, C. (2005). *Multi-country Study on Women's Health and Domestic Violence against Women Initial results on prevalence, health outcomes and women's responses.* Geneva, Switzerland: World Health Organization.

García-Moreno, C. Pallitto, C. Devries, K., Stöckl, H., Watts, C. and Abrahams, N. (2013). *Global and regional estimates of violence against women: prevalence and health effects of intimate partner violence and non-partner sexual violence.* Geneva, Switzerland: World Health Organization.

Ghorayshi, P. (1995). The Arab world: society, culture and state by Halim Barakat *The Canadian Journal of Sociology, 20*(2), 259. doi: 10.2307/3341010

Ghubash, R., El-Rufaie, O., Zoubeidi, T. Al-Shhboul, Q.M., sabri, S.M. (2004). Profile of mental disorders among the elderly United Arab Emirates population: sociodemographic correlates, *International Journal of Geriatric Psychiatry, 19*, 344-351.

Glasser S, Tanous M, Shihab S, Goldman N, Ziv A, Kaplan G. (2011). Perinatal Depressive Symptoms Among Arab Women in Northern Israel. *Maternal and Child Health J*, 1-9.

Goldberg, D., Bridges, K., Duncan-Jones, P. and Grayson, D. Detecting anxiety and depression in general medical settings. (1988). *BMJ. 297*(6653), 897–899.

Gone, J.P., & Kirmayer, L.J. (2010). On the wisdom of considering culture and context in psychopathology. In T.Millon, R.F. Krueger & E. Simonsen (Eds.), *Contemporary directions in psychopathology*. New York, London: Guilford Press.

Grauf-Grounds, C. (1982). Language as change agent: Metaphor in the work of Jay Haley and in the parables of Jesus. *Journal of Psychology and Theology, 10,* 212-220.

Grigoriadis S, Robinson GE., (2007), Gender issues in depression. *Ann Clin Psychiatry. 19*(4), 247-55.

Gureje, O. (2004). What can we learn from a cross-national study of somatic distress? *Journal of Psychosomatic Research,* 56, 409-412.

Gureje, O., Nortje, G., Makanjuola, V., Oladeji, D. Seedat, S., Jenkins, R. (2015). The role of global traditional and complementary systems of medicine in the treatment of mental health disorders *The Lancet Psychiatry.* 2(2), 168–177.

Gureje, O., Simon, G.E., Ustun, T.B. & Goldberg, D.P. (1997). Somatization in Cross-Cultural Perspective: A World Health Organization Study in Primary Care. *The American Journal of Psychiatry, 154*(7), 989-995.

Hall, E. (1976). *Beyond Culture.* New York: Doubleday.

Hall, P. (2005). Interprofessional teamwork: Professional cultures as barriers. *Journal of Interprofessional care, 19*(S1), 188-196.

Haj-Yahia, M. (1998). Beliefs about wife beating among Palestinian women: The influence of their patriarchal beliefs. *Violence Against Women, 4,* 533-558.

Haj-Yahia, M. (2000a). The incidence of wife abuse and battering and some sociodemographic correlates as revealed by two national surveys in Palestinian society. *Journal of Family Violence, 14,* 347-374.

Haj-Yahia, M. (2000b). Wife abuse and battering in the sociocultural context of Arab society. *Family Process, 39,* 237-257.

Haj-Yahia, M. (2002). Beliefs of Jordanian women about wife-beating. *Psychology of Women Quarterly,* 26, 282-291.

Haj-Yahia, M. (2003). Beliefs about wife beating among Arab men from Israel: The influence of their patriarchal ideology. *Journal of Family Violence, 18,* 193-206.

Haj-Yahia, M., & Abdo-Kaloti, R. (2003). The rates and correlates of the exposure of Palestinian adolescents to family violence: Toward an integrative-holistic approach. *Child Abuse & Neglect, 27,* 781-806.

Haj-Yahia, M., & Uysal, A. (2008). Beliefs about wife beating among medical students from Turkey. *Journal of Family Violence,* 23, 119-113.

Haley, J. (1973). *Uncommon Therapy: The psychiatric techniques of Milton H. Erickson, M.D.* New York: Norton.

Haley, J. (1976). *Problem-solving therapy.* New York: Harper & Row.

Hamdan, A., Hawamdeh, S., Hussein A. (2008). The prevalence and correlates of depressive symptoms among Arab women in a primary health care setting. *Int J Psychiatry Med, 38*(4), 453-67.

Hamdan, A. (2009). Mental health needs of Arab women. *Health Care for Women International, 30,* 593-611.

Hamdi, E., Amin, Y. & Abou-Saleh, M. T. (1997). Problems in validating endogenous depression in the arab culture by contemporary diagnostic criteria. *Journal of Affective Disorders, 44*(2-3), 131-143.,

Hamid, H., Abu-Huleh, N.S., Sharif, S.L., Raqab, M.Z., Mas'ad, D. & Abbas, A. (2004).A Primary Care Study of the Correlates of Depressive Symptoms Among Jordanian Women. *Transcultural Psychiatry, 41*(4), 487–496. doi: 10.1177/1363461504047931

Haneck, R.P. and Kibler, C.T. (1984). The role of imagery, analogy and instantiation in proverb comprehension. *Journal of Psycholinguistic Research, 13*, 393-414.

Hays, R.D., Wells, K.B., Sherbourne, C.D., Rogers, W., Spritzer, K. (1995). Functioning and well-being outcomes of patients with depression compared with chronic general medical illnesses. *Arch Gen Psychiatry* 52(1), 11–19.

Heise, L., Ellsberg, M. & Gottemoeller, M. (1999). *Ending violence against women.* Population Report, L(11).

Heise L., Pitanguy, J., & Germain, A. (1994). Violence against women: The hidden health burden. *World Bank Discussion Papers #255.* Washington D.C.: World Bank.

Hijab, N. (1996). Women and work in the Arab world. In S. Sabbagh (Ed.), *Arab women: Between defiance and restraint.* New York: Olive Branch Press.

Hinton, D.E., Lewis-Fernandez, R. (2010). Idioms of distress among trauma survivors: subtypes and clinical utility. *Culture, Medicine and Psychiatry.* doi: 10.1007/s11013-010-9175-x.

Holosko, M.J. (2001). Overview of qualitative research methods. In B.A. Thyer (Ed.), *The handbook of social research methods.* Sage Publication.

Hofmann, S.G., Sawyer, A.T., Witt, A.A. and Oh, D. (2010). The Effect of Mindfulness-Based Therapy on Anxiety and Depression: A Meta-Analytic Review. *J Consult Clin Psychol.* 78(2), 169–183. doi: 10.1037/a0018555.

Honor killings still tolerated. (2007, March 11). *IRIN Humanitarian News and Analysis.* (Human Rights Watch interview with Asma Khader, Amman, July 12, 2003).

Ibrahim, A-S and Ibrahim, R.M. (1993). Is psychotherapy really needed in nonwestern cultures? The case of Arab countries. *Psychological Reports, 72*, 881-882. doi: 10.2466/pr0.1993.72.3.881

Inter-Israeli Task Force on Israeli Arab Issues. Retrieved from iataskforce.org. http://www.iataskforce.org/issues/view/2#sthash.tsQFDUfV.dpuf

Jones, A. Gendercide Watch 1999-2013.

Jones, S.D., Ehiri, J., Anyanwu E. (2004). Female genital mutilation in developing countries: an agenda for public health response. *Eur. J.Obstet. Gynecol. Reprod. Biology, 116*, 144–151.

Joseph, S. (1994). Brother/Sister relationships: Connectivity, love, and power in the reproduction of patriarchy in Lebanon. In S. Hopkins, & Ibrahim,

Saad Eddin (Eds.), *Arab Society: Class, Gender, Power, and Development*. The American University in Cairo Press.

Joseph, S. (1996). Patriarchy and development in the Arab world. *Gender and Development*, 4(2), 14-19.

Katon, W., Kleinman, A. & Rosen, G. (1982). Depression and somatization. *The American Journal of Medicine*, 72, 127-135; 241-247.

Katon, W., Ries, R. & Kleinman, A. (1984). The prevalence of somatization in primary care. *Comprehensive psychiatry*, 25, 208-215.

Kessler, R. C., Berglund, P., Demler, O., Jin, R., Koretz, D., Merikangas, K. R., & Wang, P. S. (2003). The epidemiology of major depressive disorder: results from the National Comorbidity Survey Replication (NCS-R). *Jama*, 289(23), 3095-3105.

Khalife, N. (2010, January 29). Dubai's shameful record on rape *The Guardian* UK.

Khalifa, N., Hardie, T., Latif, S., Jamil, I., & Walker, D. M. (2011). Beliefs about Jinn, black magic and the evil eye among Muslims: age, gender and first language influences. *International Journal of Culture and Mental Health*, 4(1), 68-77.

Khasawne, O., Hijazi, A.K.Y., Salman, N.H., (2011). Polygamy and its impact on the upbringing of children: A Jordanian perspective. *Journal of Comparative Family Studies*, 42(4), 563-577.

Kilzieh, N., Rastam, S., Maziak, W. and Ward, K.D., (2008). Comorbidity of depression with chronic diseases: A population-based study in Aleppo, Syria. *Int J Psychiatry Med.*, 38(2), 169–184.

Kilzieh N., Rastam, S., Ward, K.D., Maziak, W., (2010). Gender, depression and physical impairment: an epidemiologic perspective from Aleppo, Syria. *Soc Psychiatry Psychiatr Epidemiol*, 45(6), 595-602. doi: 10.1007/s00127-009-0076-7

Kinrys, G., Wygant, L.E. (2005). Anxiety disorders in women: does gender matter to treatment? *Review Bras Psiquiatr, 27(II)*, S43-50.

Kirmayer, L.J. (1984). Culture, affect and somatization, Part I. *Transcultural Psychiatry Research Review*, *21*, 159-188.

Kirmayer, L.J. (1992). The body's insistence on meaning: Metaphor as presentation and representation in illness experience. *Medical Anthropology Quarterly*, 6(4), 323-346.

Kirmayer, L.J. (1994). Improvisation and authority in illness meaning, *Culture, Medicine and Psychiatry*, *18*, 183-214.

Kirmayer, L.J. (2003). Asklepian dreams: The ethos of the wounded-healer in the clinical encounter. *Transcultural Psychiatry*, 40(2), 248-277.

Kirmayer, L.J. (2004). The cultural diversity of healing: meaning, metaphor and mechanism. *British Medical Bulletin*, *69*, 33-48.

Kirmayer, L.J. (2006). Beyond the 'New Cross-Cultural Psychiatry': Cultural biology, discursive psychology and the ironies of globalization. *Transcultural Psychiatry, 43*(1), 126-144. doi: 10.1177/1363461506061761

Kirmayer, L.J. (2007). Celan's poetics of Alterity. *Monash Bioethics Review, 26*(4), 21-35.

Kirmayer, L.J. (2008). Empathy and alterity in cultural psychiatry. *Ethos, 30*(4), 457-474.

Kirmayer, L.J. (2013). 50 years of transcultural psychiatry. *Transcultural Psychiatry, 50*(1), 3-5.

Kirmayer, L.J., Robbins, J. M., Dworkind, M. & Yaffe, M.J. (1993). Somatization and the recognition of depression and anxiety in primary care. *American Journal of Psychiatry, 150*(5), 34-739.

Kirmayer, L. J., Young, A. (1998). Culture and somatization: Clinical epidemiological, and ethnographic perspectives. *Psychosomatic Medicine, 60*, 420-430. doi: 0033-3174/98/6004-0420

Kishor, S. (2005). *Violence against women: A statistical overview, challenges and gaps in data collection and methodology and approaches for overcoming them.* Geneva: UN Division for the Advancement of Women in collaboration with Economic Commission for Europe (ECE) and World Health Organization (WHO).

Kleinman, A. (1982). Neurasthenia and depression: a study of somatization and culture in China. *Culture, medicine and psychiatry, 6*(2), 117-190.

Kleinman, A. & Kleinman, J. (1985). Somatization: the interconnections in Chinese society among culture, depressive experiences, and the meaning of pain. In A. Kleinman, & B. Good (Eds.), *Culture and Depression.* Berkeley: University of California Press.

Kohrt, B. A., & Hruschka, D. J. (2010). Nepali concepts of psychological trauma: the role of idioms of distress, ethnopsychology and ethnophysiology in alleviating suffering and preventing stigma. *Culture, Medicine, and Psychiatry,34*(2), 322-352.

Kohrt, B.A., Rasmussen, A., Kaiser, B.N. Haroz, E.E., Maharjan, S.M., Mutamba, B.B., de Jong, J.TVM and Hinton, D.E. (2014). Cultural concepts of distress and psychiatric disorders: literature review and research recommendations for global mental health epidemiology. *International Journal of Epidemiology,43*, 365–406. doi:10.1093/ije/dyt227

Koran, Sura 4, Chapter 3.

Kopp, R., (1995). *Metaphor Therapy: Using Client-generated Metaphors in Psychotherapy.* New York, NY: Brunner-Routledge.

Kramer, M. (1996). *Arab Awakening and Islamic Revival: The Politics of Ideas in the Middle East.* New Brunswick, NJ: Transaction Publishers.

Kramer, M. (1993). Arab Nationalism: Mistaken Identity. *Daedalus*, Summer, 171-206. Retrieved from http://www.geocities.com/martinkramerorg/ArabNationalism.htm

Krishnan, M. (2012, April 20). Female infanticide in India mocks claims of progress, *DW*.

Lamanna, M. A., Riedmann, A., & Stewart, S. (2014). *Marriages, families, and relationships: Making choices in a diverse society*. Cengage Learning.

Lasebikan, V.O., Ejidokun, A., Coker, O.A. (2012). Prevalence of mental disorders and profile of disablement among primary health care service users in Lagos Island. *Epidemiology Research International*, 2-6. doi: 10.1155/2012/357348.

Lavee, Y., McCubbin, H. & Olson, D. (1987). The effect of stressful life event and transitions on family functioning and well-being. *Journal of Marriage and the Family, 49*, 857-873.

Leighton, A. H. (1959). *My name is legion: The Stirling County Study I*. New York: Basic Books.

Leff, J. P. (1973). Culture and the differentiation of emotional states. *The British Journal of Psychiatry, 123*(574), 299-306.

Lev-Wiesel, R. & Al-Krenawi, A. (1999). Attitude towards marriage and marital quality: A comparison among Israeli Arabs differentiated by religion. *Family Relations, 48*(1), 51-56.

Lewis, Bernard (2004). *The Crisis of Islam*. New York City: Random House.

Lim, A., Hoek, H. & Blom, J. (2014). The attribution of psychotic symptoms to jinn in Islamic patients. *Transcultural Psychiatry, 0*(0), 1-15.

Lipowski, Z.J. (1984). What does the word 'psychosomatic' really mean? A historical and semantic inquiry. *Psychosomatic Medicine, 46*(2). doi: 0033-3174/84.

Lipowski, Z.J. (1988). Somatization. The concept and its clinical application. *The American Journal of Psychiatry, 145*, 1358-1368.

Lobo, A., Garcia-Campayo, S., Campos, R., et al. (1996). Somatization in primary care in Spain: I. Estimates of prevalence and clinical characteristics. *British Journal of Psychiatry, 168*, 344-348.

Alan D Lopez, Colin D Mathers,Majid Ezzati,Dean T Jamison, Christopher J L MurrayLopez, Mathers, Ezzati, Jamison & Murray (2006). Global and regional burden of disease and risk factors, 2001: systematic analysis of population health data. *Lancet, 367*, 1747–57.

Luthar, S. (Ed.). (2003). *Resilience and Vulnerability: Adaptation in the context of childhood adversities*. New York: Cambridge University Press.

Luthar, S.S., Cicchetti, D., Becker, B. (2000). The construct of resilience: a critical evaluation and guidelines for future work. *Child Dev. 71*(3), 543-62.

Mahler, M. (1968). *On human symbiosis and the vicissitudes of individuation: Infantile psychosis* (Volume 1). New York: International Universities Press.

Mahler, M., Bergman, A. and Pine, F. (1975). *The psychological birth of the infant: Symbiosis and individuation*. New York: Basic Books.

Malatesta, V. J. (2007). Introduction: The need to address older women's mental health issues. *Journal of women & aging, 19*(1-2), 1-12.

Manji, I. (2011). *Allah, Liberty and Love: The Courage to Reconcile Faith and Freedom*. New York: Free Press.

Mass, M., & Al-Krenawi, A. (1994). When a man encounters a woman, Satan is also present: On professional encounters in Bedouin society. *Society and Welfare, 14*(2), 181-197.

Matthews, K., Wing. R., Kuller, L. (1990). Influences of natural menopause on psychological characteristics and symptoms of middle-aged healthy women. *Journal of Consulting and Clinical Psychology, 58*, 345–363.

Mazher, M., I, Abbas, T, (2011). *Honour, Violence, Women and Islam*. Routledge, New York.

Maziak, W., & Asfar, T. (2003). Physical abuse in low income women in Aleppo, Syria. *Health Care for Women International, 24*, 313–26.

Mayou, R., Kirmayer, L.J., Simon, G., Kroenke, K., Sharpe, M. (2005). Somatoform disorders: Time for a new approach in DSM-V. *American Journal of Psychiatry, 162*(5), 847-855.

McCormick, K., Stricklin S,, Nowak, T. and Rous, B. (2008).Using eco-mapping to understand family strengths and resources. *Young Exceptional Children, 12*(1), 17-28.

Mernissi, F. (1975). *Beyond the veil: Male-female dynamic in modern Muslim society*. London: Schendman.

Messiri, R. (1984). *The Egyptian Personality: Through the Egyptian Folklore*. Cairo: Al-Heah Al-Messriah Llketab (in Arabic).

Metaphor. (n.d.). In Online Etymology Dictionary. Retrieved from http://www.etymonline.com/index.php?term=metaphor

Mezzich, J.E., Salloum, I.M.,Cloninger, C. R., Salvador-Carulla. (2010). Person-centred Integrative Diagnosis: Conceptual Bases and Structural Model. *Canadian Journal of Psychiatry, 55*(11), 705.

Mickus, M., & Colenda, C. (2000). Knowledge of mental health benefits and provider preference. *Psychiatric Services, 51*, 199-203.

Miller, I.W., Epstein, N.B., Bishop, D.S. & Keitner, G.I. (1985). The McMaster Family Assessment Device: Reliability and validity. *Journal of Marital and Family Therapy, 11*, 345-356.

Milner, Larry S. (2000). *Hardness of Heart/Hardness of Life: The Stain of Human Infanticide*. University Press of America.

Mirza, I., & Jenkins, R. (2004). Risk factors, prevalence, and treatment of anxiety and depressive disorders in Pakistan: systematic review. *Bmj,328*(7443), 794.

Morse, D.S., Dgbary, S.S., Paldi, Y.,& Clark, C.J. (2012). An effect that is deeper than beating: Family violence in Jordanian women. *Families, Systems & Health, 30*(1), 19-31.

Morrison, Z. (2007). Caring about Sexual Assault: The Effects of Sexual Assault on Families, and the Effects on Victim/Survivors of Family Responses to Sexual Assault [online]. *Family Matters, 76*: 55-63.

Mullick, M. S., Khalifa, N., Nahar, J. S., & Walker, D. M. (2013). Beliefs about Jinn, black magic and evil eye in Bangladesh: the effects of gender and level of education. *Mental Health, Religion & Culture, 16*(7), 719-729.

Murray C.J.L. and Lopez, A.D. (1996). *The global burden of disease: A comprehensive assessment of mortality and disability from diseases, injuries and risk factors in 1990 and projected to 2020. Worldwide, mental disorders inflict tremendous morbidity, mortality, and impairment.* Cambridge: Harvard University Press.

National Research Council and Institute of Medicine (2009). *Preventing mental, emotional, and behavioral disorders among young people: progress and possibilities.* Washington, DC: The National Academic Press.

Nichter, M. (1981). Idioms of distress: Alternatives in the expression of psychosocial distress: A case study from South India. *Culture, Medicine and Psychiatry,* 5, 379-408. doi: 0165-005X/81/0054-0379.

Nichter, M. (2008). Coming to our senses: Appreciating the sensorial in medical anthropology. *Transcultural Psychiatry,* 45(2), 163-197. doi: 10.1177/1363461508089764.

Nichter, M. (2010). Idioms of distress revisited. *Cultural Medical Psychiatry, 34,* 401-416.

Nguyen, D.L. (1969). *Four-syllable idiomatic expressions in Vietnamese.* Honolulu: East-West Center.

Nguyen N., Foulks, E.F., Carlin, K. (1991). Proverbs as psychological interpretations among Vietnamese. *Asian Folklore Studies, 50,* 311-318.

Norrick, N.R. (1985). How proverbs mean: Sematic studies in English proverbs. New York: Mouton.

Norton, R.W. (1981). Soft magic. In Wilder-Mott & J.H. Weakland (Eds.), *Rigor and imagination: Essays from the legacy of Gregory Bateson* (pp. 299-320). New York: Praeger.

Novosti R. (2008, November 11). Average Arab reads 4 pages a year. *Sputnik News*. Retrieved from: sputniknews.com/world/20081111/118255514.html#ixzz3S7hDgMow

Nye, R. (2005). Review paper of: Idioms of distress: Psychosomatic disorders in medical and imaginative literature by Lilian R. Furst. *Comparative Literature Studies,* 42(3), 244-246.

Obeid,N., Chang,D.F. and Ginges, J. (2010). Beliefs About Wife Beating: An Exploratory Study With Lebanese Students. *Violence Against Women, 16*(6), 691-712.

Ohaeri, J.U. & Odejide, O.A. (1994). Somatization symptoms among patients using primary health care facilities in a rural community in Nigeria. *The American Journal of Psychiatry, 15*, 728-731.

Okasha, A., Bishry, Z., Khalil, A. H., Darwish, T. A., El Dawla, A. S., & Shohdy, A. (1994). Panic disorder. An overlapping or independent entity? *The British Journal of Psychiatry, 164*(6), 818-825.

Okasha, A., Karam, E. (1998). Mental health services and research in the Arab world. *Acta Psychiatrica Scandanavia*, 98, 406-413.

Okasha, A., Maj, M. eds. (2001). *Images in Psychiatry: An Arab Perspective*. Cairo, Egypt: Scientific Book House.

Orthony, A., Reynolds, R.E. & Alter, J.A. (1978). Metaphor: Theoretical and empirical research. *Psychological Bulletin, 85*, 919-943.

Osman, O.T. and Al-Radi, O. (2005).The influence of culture and religion on mental health treatment: A stigma revisited. *WIAMH Newsletter, 2*(20), 19.

Paykel, E.S. (1991). Depression in women. *Br J Psychiatry Suppl,10*, 22-9.

Pateman, C. (1988). *The Sexual Contract*. Stanford University Press.

Pelham, L. (2014, August 3). Israel's Secret Honor Killings, *The Daily Beast*.

Peratis, K. (2004). Honoring the killers: Justice denied for 'honor' crimes in Jordan. *Human Rights Watch, 16*(1E).

Pew Research Center (2011). *Executive Summary: The Future of the Global Muslim Population*.

PUCL Report (1982). *People's Union for Civil Liberties*. Delhi, India.

Qazi, F. (2014, June 30). America's Honor Killings a growing reality. *Islamic Monthly*. Retrieved from http://theislamicmonthly.com/americas-honor-killings-a-growing-reality/

Radford, M., Nakane, Y., Ohta, Y., Mann, L., & Kalucy, R. (1989). A study of depression in two cultures: A transcultural study with Japanese and Australian clinically depressed patients. *Psychiatry and Clinical Neurosciences, 43*(2), 119-132.

Racy, J. (1980). Somatization in Saudi women: A therapeutic challenge. *British Journal of Psychiatry, 137*, 212-216.

Ridenour, T.A., Daley, J.G. & Reich, W. (1999). Factor analyses of the Family Assessment Device. *Family Process, 38*(4), 497-510.

Rodgers-Farmen, A.Y. & Potocky-Tripody, M. (2001). Gender, ethnicity and race matter. In B.A. Thyer (Ed.), *The handbook of social research methods*. Sage.

Sa'ar, A. and Younis, Y. (2010). Masculinity in crisis: The case of Palestinians Israel. In Z.S. Salhi (Ed.), Gender and Diversity in the Middle East and North Africa (pp. 13-32). Oxon and New York: Routledge.

Sadiqi, F., (2014). Gender and violence in Muslim societies: Patriarchy, Islamism and politics in the Middle East and North Africa, *Gender and Development*, 22(1), 185-187.

Saint Arnault, D., Kim, O. (2008). Is there an Asian idiom of distress? Somatic symptoms in female Japanese and Korean students. *Archives of Psychiatric Nursing*, 22(1), 27-38.

Salem, M.O. (2014). Suggested avenues to reduce the stigma of mental illness in the Middle East. *Int J Soc Psychiatry*. doi: 10.1177/0020764014537234

Salem-Pickartz, J.A. (2015). Mental Health: Arab States. In *Encyclopedia of Women & Islamic Cultures*. Retrieved from http://referenceworks.brillonline.com/entries/encyclopedia-of-women-and-islamic-cultures/mental-health-arab-states-EWICCOM_0184b.

Salhi, Z.S. (2010). (Ed.). *Gender and Diversity in the Middle East and North Africa*. Oxon and New York: Routledge.

Salhi, Z.S. (2013). (Ed.). *Gender and Violence in Islamic Societies*, London and New York: I.B. Tauris & Co Ltd.

Salloum, I.M. and Mezzich, J.E. (2009). *Psychiatric Diagnosis: Challenges and Prospects*. UK: Wiley and Sons.

Savaya, R. (1995). Attitudes towards family and marital counseling among Israeli Arab women. *Journal of Social Service Research*, 21(1), 35-51.

Sayed, M.A. (2002). Arabic psychiatry and psychology: The physician who is a philosopher and the physician who is not a philosopher: some cultural considerations. *Social Behavior and Personality*, *30*(3), 235-242.

Seligman, M. E. P. (1975). *Helplessness: On Depression, Development, and Death*. San Francisco: W. H. Freeman.

Shalhoub-Kevorkian, N. (1997). Wife abuse: A method of social control. *Israel Social Science Research*, *12*(1), 59-72.

Shapiro, S.L. and Carlson, L.E. (2009). *The art and science of mindfulness: Integrating mindfulness into psychology and the helping professions*. Washington DC, US: American Psychological Association. http://dx.doi.org/10.1037/11885-000

Shidhaye, R., Mendenhall, E., Sumathipala, K., Sumathipala, A. Patel, V. (2013). Association of somatoform disorders with anxiety and depression in women in low- and middle-income countries: A systematic review. *International Review of Psychiatry*, 23(1), 65-76.

Shoup, J. (2001). *Ethnic Groups of Africa and the Middle East: An Encyclopedia*. CA: ABC Clio.

Shweder, R.A. (1991). *Thinking through Cultures: Expeditions in Cultural Psychology*, Cambridge, MA: Harvard University Press.

Seedat, S., Scott, K.M., Angermeyer, M.C., Berglund, P., Bromet, E.J., Brugha, T.S., Demyttenaere, K., de Girolamo, G., Haro, J.M., Jin, R., Karam, E.G., Kovess-Masfety, V., Levinson, D., Medina, Mora, M.E. , Ormel, O.Y., Pennell, J. Posada-Villa, J., Sampson, N.A., Williams, D., Kessler, R.C. (2009). Cross-national associations between gender and mental disorders in the World Health Organization World Mental Health Surveys. *Arch Gen Psychiatry*. 66(7), 785-95. doi: 10.1001/archgenpsychiatry.2009.36

Shouby E (1951). The influence of Arabic language on the Psychology of the Arabs. *Middle East Journal* 5, 284.

Sikseck, A. (2014). *Open Letter to Enlightened Muslim Leaders*, Facebook.

Sorensen S, Pinquart, M, Duberstein, P. (2002). How effective are interventions with caregivers? An updated meta-analysis. *Gerontologist*, 42(3), 356–372.

Sontag, S. (1978). *Illness as a metaphor* (1st ed.). Farrar, Straus and Giroux.

Spataro, J.,Mullen, P.E.,Burgess, P.M., Wells, D.L., Moss, S.A. (2004). Impact of child sexual abuse on mental health. *The British Journal of Psychiatry*. May, 1-16. doi: 10.1192/bjp.184.5.416.

Stelter, R. The transformation of body experience into language. (2000) *Journal of Phenomenological Psychology*, *31*(1), 63-77.

Strauss, Gregg, (2012). Is Polygamy Inherently Unequal? *Ethics*, *122*(3), 516-544.

Strine T.W. and Hootman, J.M. (2007). US national prevalence and correlates of low back and neck pain among adults. *Arthritis Care & Research*, 57(4), 656–665.

Sullivan-Norton, C. (1985). The therapeutic functions of metaphor. *Journal of Communication Therapy*, 4, 138-163.

Sullivan, C. (1986). *The enthymematic structure of metaphor*. Paper presented to the International Conference on Argumentation, Amsterdam.

Tappis H., Biermann, E., Glass, N., Tilevab, M. and Shannon Doocy, (2012). Domestic Violence Among Iraqi Refugees in Syria. *Health Care for Women International*, 33(3), 285-297.

The Times of India (2013, September 1). Dowry deaths: One woman dies every hour.

The Islamic Monthly (2014, June 30). Qazi, Farhana. America's honor killings a growing reality. theislamicmonthly.com/americas-honor-killings-a-growing-reality/

Thomas, C.K., Hook, E. (2009). *Leila Ahmed*. Regents of the University of Minnesota.

Timimi, S.B., (1995). Adolescence in immigrant Arab families. *Psychotherapy: Theory, Research, Practice, Training*, 32(1), 141-149.

Tiziana, L., Coast, E., Narayanan, S. and de Graft Aikins, A. (2012). Diabetes and depression comorbidity and socio-economic status in low and middle income countries (LMICs): A mapping of the evidence. *Globalization and Health*, 8(39). doi:10.1186/1744-8603-8-3

To break the pentameter that was the first. (n.d.). In *Columbia World of Quotations*. Retrieved from http://quotes.dictionary.com/To_break_the_pentameter_that_was_the_first

Tseng, W.S. and McDermot, J.F. (1981). *Culture, Mind and Therapy*. New York: Bruner/Mazel.

Tuncer, C. (1995). Mental Illness in an Islamic Mediterranean Culture: Turkey.

In Al Issa (Ed.), *Handbook of culture and mental illness: An international perspective* (pp. 169-172). International Universities Press, USA.

Tutty, L.M., Rothery, M.A. and Grinnell, R.M. (1996). *Qualitative Research for Social Workers*. Boston: Allyn and Bacon.

Ungar, M. (2010). What is resilience across cultures and contexts? Advances to the theory of positive development among individuals and families under stress. *Journal of Family Psychotherapy, 21*, 1-16.

United Nations Development Fund Report (UNDF) (2006). The Rise of Women in the Arab World.

United Nations Development Fund Report (UNDF) (2008). Retrieved from http://pun.sagepub.com/content/16/4/406.refs

UN Habitat (2006). *State of the World's Cities: Trends in Sub-Saharan Africa.*

Ungar, M. (2011). The social ecology of resilience: Addressing contextual and cultural ambiguity of a nascent construct. *American Journal of Orthopsychiatry, 81*(1), 1-17.

Ungar, M. (2013). (Ed.) *The Social Ecology of* Resilience. New York, Heidelberg, Dordrecht, London: Springer.

University of Cambridge News. (2013, June 2013). Belief that honour killings are justified still prevalent among Jordan's next generation. http://www.cam.ac.uk/research/news/belief-that-honour-killings-are-justified-still-prevalent-among-jordans-next-generation-study-shows.

Van der Kwaak, A. (1992) Female circumcision and gender identity: A questionable alliance? *Social Science & Medicine,* 35(6), 777-787.

Van Duijl, M., Nijenhuis, E., Komproe, I.H., Hajo, B.P.E., Gernaat, and de Jong, J.T. (2010). Dissociative Symptoms and Reported Trauma Among Patients with Spirit Possession and Matched Healthy Controls in Uganda. *Cult Med Psychiatry. 34(2),* 380–400. doi: 10.1007/s11013-010-9171-PMCID: PMC2878595.

Wang, P.S., Aguilar-Gaxiola, Alonso, Angermeyer, Borges, Bromet, Bruffaerts, de Girlolamo, de Graaf, Gureje, Haro, Karam, Kessler, Kovess, Lane, Lee, Levinson, Ono, Petukhova, Posada-Villa, Seedat, & Wells. (2007). Worldwide use of mental health services for anxiety, mood, and substance disorders: results from 17 countries in the WHO World Mental Health (WMH) Surveys. *Lancet. 370,* 841–850.

Wang, P.S., Angermeyer, M., Borges, G., Bruffaerts, R., Chiu, W.T., de Girolamo, G., Fayyad, J., Gureje, O., Haro, J.M., Huang, H., Kessler, R.C., Kovess, V., Levinson, D., Nakane, Y., Brown, M.A. Ormel, J.H., Posada-Villa, J., Aguilar-Gaxiola, S., Alonso, J., Sing Lee, S., Heeringa, P., Chatterji S. and Ustun, T.B. (2007). Delay and failure in treatment seeking after first onset of mental disorders in the World Health Organization's World Mental Health Survey Initiative. *World Psychiatry.* 6(3), 177–185.

Watzlawick, P. (1978). *The language of change: Elements of therapeutic communication.* New York: Basic Books.

Wei, L., Mayouf, M.A. (2009). The effects of the social status of the elderly in Libya on the way they institutionally interact and communicate with younger physicians. *Journal of Pragmatics, 41*, 136-146.

Weiss, M.G., Raguram, R., and Channabasavanna, S.M. (1995). Cultural dimensions of psychiatric diagnosis. A comparison of DSM-III-R and illness explanatory models in south India. *Br J Psychiatry, 166(3)*, 353-9.

Wells, K.B., Golding, J.M., Burnam, and M.A. (1988) Psychiatric disorder and limitations in physical functioning in a sample of the Los Angeles general population. *Am J Psychiatry 145*(6), 712–717.

Weissman, J. and Levine, S. (2007). Anxiety Disorders and Older Women. In Malatesta (Ed.), *Mental Health Issues of Older Women: A Comprehensive Review for Health Care Professionals* (pp.79-102). Haworth Press.

Werbner, P. (2007). Veiled interventions in pure space: Honour, shame and embodied struggles among Muslims. *Theory Culture Society, 24*, 161-186.

Werner, E.E. and Smith, R.S. (2005). *Research, Policy, and Practice in Children's Mental Health. 19*(1), 11-14

West, J. (1987). Psychotherapy in the Eastern province of Saudi Arabia. *Psychotherapy, 24(1)*, 105-107.

Whaley, B.B. (1993). When 'Try, try again' turns to 'You're beating a dead horse': The rhetorical characteristics of proverbs and their potential for influencing therapeutic change. *Metaphor and Symbolic Activity, 8(2)*, 127-139.

Whiting, B.J. (1932). The nature of proverbs. *Harvard Studies and Notes in Philology and Literature, 14*, 273-307.

Witztum, E., Van Der Hart, O., Friedman, B. (1988). The use of metaphors in psychotherapy. *Journal of Contemporary Psychotherapy*, 1-11.

World Health Organization (1993). Retrieved from http://www.who.int/mental_health/publications/women_mh_evidence_review/en/

World Health Organization (2000). *Women's mental health: an evidence based review.* Geneva: World Health Organization. Retrieved from www.who.int

World Health Organization (2007). *Women, ageing and health: a framework for action: focus on gender.* Geneva: World Health Organization.

World Health Organization (2008). Retrieved from http://www.who.int/healthinfo/global_burden_disease/2004_report_update/en/

World Bank, (2010). *Defining civil society.* Retrieved from http://go.worldbank.org/4CE7W046K0

World Health Organization (2013). *WHO Traditional Medicine Strategy 2014–2023.* Geneva: World Health Organization.

Yap, P.M. (1951). Mental diseases peculiar to certain cultures: A survey of comparative psychiatry. *Journal of Mental Science, 97*, 313-327

Zeig, J.K. (1995). Experiential approaches to clinician development. In Zeig (Ed.), *The evolution of psychotherapy: The third conference*. New York: Brunner/Mazel.

Zuniga, M.E. (1991). 'Dichos' as metaphorical tools for resistant Latino clients. *Psychotherapy, 28*, 480-483.

Zuniga, M.E. (1992). Using metaphors in therapy: Dichos and Latino clients. *Social Work, 37*, 55-60.

Index

Note: Page locators in *italic* refer to tables.

www.ingramcontent.com/pod-product-compliance
Lightning Source LLC
LaVergne TN
LVHW011802200926
848484LV00003B/760